OUTCOME-ORIENTED REHABILITATION

Principles, Strategies, and Tools for Effective Program Management

Edited by

Pat Kitchell Landrum, MA, CCC

President
Rehab Results: Consultants in Rehabilitation Technology
and Organizational Change
Grand Junction, Colorado

Nancy D. Schmidt, MS

Vice President of Specialty Programs
New England Rehabilitation Hospital
Woburn, Massachusetts

Alvin McLean, Jr., PhD

Senior Vice President
Paradigm Health Corporation
Concord, California

Endicott College
Beverly, Mass. 01915

AN ASPEN PUBLICATION®
Aspen Publishers, Inc.
Gaithersburg, Maryland
1995

Library of Congress Cataloging-in-Publication Data

Outcome-oriented rehabilitation: principles, strategies, and tools for effective program management
[edited by] Pat Kitchell Landrum, Nancy D. Schmidt, Alvin McLean, Jr.
p.   cm.
Includes bibliographical references and index.
ISBN 0-8342-0665-X (printed casebound: alk. paper)
1. Medical rehabilitation. 2. Hospitals—Rehabilitation services.
I. Landrum, Pat Kitchell. II. Schmidt, Nancy D. III. McLean, Alvin.

RM930.093   1995
362.1'786'068—dc20
95-12372
CIP

Editorial Resources: Lenda Hill

Library of Congress Catalog Card Number: 95-12372
ISBN: 0-8342-0665-X

Printed in the United States of America

1 2 3 4 5

Table of Contents

List of Contributors

EDITORS

Pat Kitchell Landrum, MA, CCC
President
Rehab Results: Consultants in
    Rehabilitation Technology and
    Organizational Change
Grand Junction, Colorado

Nancy D. Schmidt, MS
Vice President of Specialty
    Programs
New England Rehabilitation Hospital
Woburn, Massachusetts

Alvin McLean, Jr., PhD
Senior Vice President
Paradigm Health Corporation
Concord, California

AUTHORS

Ann Bodin
Paradigm Health Corporation
Concord, California

Ernest T. Bryant, PhD, ABCN
Director, Head Trauma and
    Neuropsychology Services
Kaiser Permanente Medical Group
Kaiser Foundation Rehabilitation
    Center
Vallejo, California

Laura E. Cayce, PT, MHA
Vice President, General Manager
    Persona Care
TheraTx, Inc.
Atlanta, Georgia

D. Nathan Cope, MD
Senior Vice President, Medical
    Affairs
Chief Medical Officer
Paradigm Health Corporation
Concord, California

Gerben DeJong, PhD
Director
National Rehabilitation Hospital
    Research Center
Director
Research and Training Center on
    Medical Rehabilitation Services
    and Health Policy
Medlantic Research Institute
Professor
Department of Family Medicine
Georgetown University School of
    Medicine
Washington, DC

Randall W. Evans, PhD
Senior Vice President
Learning Services Corporation
Durham, North Carolina
Clinical Associate Professor
Department of Psychiatry
UNC Medical School
Chapel Hill, North Carolina

Joseph D. Friedman, MA
Principal, Managing Director
The Clarion Group
Mill Valley, California

William J. Haffey, PhD
Vice President, Clinical Services
TheraTx, Inc.
Atlanta, Georgia

Louis E. Hallman, III
Vice President, Corporate
    Development
TheraTx, Inc.
Atlanta, Georgia

Richard D. Hansen, MS, MSW
Medical Group Management
    Association
Englewood, Colorado

J. Scott Ling, PsyD
Coordinator, Neurobehavioral
    Services
Learning Services Corporation
Durham, North Carolina

John O'Lear, MBA
Chief Operating Officer
Paradigm Health Corporation
Concord, California

Michael D. Peters, PhD
Paradigm Health Corporation
Concord, California

**Paul A. Repicky, PhD, MA/LS,
    MAT**
Chief Executive Officer and
    Chairman
ProStrat, Inc.
Del Mar, California

Leslie Small, MS, MEd
Program Director
Learning Services Corporation
Durham, North Carolina

Paula Sundance, MD
Vice President, Medical Affairs
Paradigm Health Corporation
Concord, California
Director, Regional Rehabilitation
The Permanente Medical Group
Vallejo, California

Janet P. Sutton, PhD
Senior Research Associate
National Rehabilitation Hospital
    Research Center
Medlantic Research Institute
Washington, DC

Brian D. Vervynck
Senior Vice President
Strategic Partnerships
Paradigm Health Corporation
Concord, California

Preface

PURPOSE AND INTENDED RESULTS

The first purpose of this book is to provide managers in rehabilitation with a model and a road map that link key principles and practices found in successful businesses to the work of managing rehabilitation services. The second purpose is to inspire rehabilitationists to take a stand to transform the industry as we move into the next millennium.

In *Outcome-Oriented Rehabilitation*, we will examine what has been shown to be effective in leading businesses and demonstrate how these principles translate to the rehabilitation environment. We will provide specific tools for measuring the efficacy of management principles including: patient outcome achievement, fiscal stability, and profitability, as well as satisfaction among all customers served. This book is designed as a working tool for managers and providers of rehabilitation. Our intended result is that readers will apply the concepts presented in their own work setting at general to very specific levels. Readers will be able to demonstrate the results applying these ideas to their colleagues, superiors, direct reports, and of customers in a measurable fashion.

For many of the authors, the writing was more difficult than we expected. We were breaking new ground as we looked toward rehabilitation in the next millennium. We drew on our beliefs and experiences to get to the "kernel of truth," took a stand for producing an outcome worth achieving, and were accountable for producing that result. We had to challenge our own beliefs in the face of our commitment to make this a functional working tool for our customers. We then applied a data-driven approach to operationalize our hypotheses. In this regard, the book expresses the feelings that many rehabilitation providers face each day:

the feelings of commitment and accountability. Rehabilitation is fundamentally about making a difference in the lives of those we serve as a result of specific intervention at specific points in time. It is the work of human beings. The compelling nature of rehabilitation, given the crucial difference that can be made, is that it is an elegant opportunity to demonstrate the highest level of customer service. We must be responsible to our customers if we are to make a difference in their lives and the lives of those around them.

This is not an empirical book, but a book of principles and distinctions. You will notice as you read the text and references that we have borrowed from other disciplines to try to expand on our understanding of the business of rehabilitation. We invite you to use the book to challenge your assumptions, your thinking, your routines, and your practices.

HOW TO USE THIS BOOK

The first half of *Outcome-Oriented Rehabilitation* defines clinical outcome and principles for achieving target results at several levels of the rehabilitation continuum from medical instability to community and home integration. The second half presents key business practices that will support providers in delivering on their commitments. Overall, the book is for direct application in the transformation of rehabilitation to meet the managed health care challenge of today and to take rehabilitation into the next millennium.

You, the reader, may choose to target specific topics in the book that you see needed in your immediate context or to read the book as a whole. We suggest that however you choose to read, prior to reading each chapter you clarify what outcome you want and how you plan to use your new knowledge or insight. The degree to which one is committed to a result directly impacts the degree to which that outcome is achieved. We would like you to practice this principle in your reading of *Outcome-Oriented Rehabilitation*.

We invite you to contact us if we can be of service as you move to transform your individual performance and your business into an outcome-oriented rehabilitation service system.

Pat Kitchell Landrum
Nancy D. Schmidt
Alvin McLean, Jr.

Acknowledgments

Writing this book has been an opportunity to put our feet and our fingers where our mouths were. We are grateful for the gracious listening we have been granted by so many in its making. We are humbled by the challenges our patients face each day.

Many people contributed to the development of this book, including providers, payers, and consumers of rehabilitation. Although we would like to thank them all, we will acknowledge a few who made completion of this project possible.

First, we wish to acknowledge our authors. We led the writing of this book on a "managed care" time line. Our authors were exemplars of what outcome-oriented rehabilitation is all about: they produced on task, on time, and at quality standard. We are thankful for their leadership. Our authors expressed the underlying urgency that drives rehabilitation. We thank the people who have had illnesses, injuries, and traumas requiring rehabilitation. These people are our inspiration and our teachers. We hope that this book will contribute to a better community for people with disabilities.

We would like to thank Aspen Publishers for providing customer service and for publishing this book at breakneck speed. Aspen met the urgency of this topic with extraordinary partnership and efficiency. Loretta Stock and Mary Anne Langdon were generous coaches and guides. Each team we worked with was professional, clear, and fun.

Carmella Gonella, PhD was a powerful partner in this venture. As our field reviewer, she gave us much needed guidance, validation, and editorial support. She, too, demonstrated what this book is about by being true to her word and challenging our thinking. Her leadership and innovation in the field of rehabilitation were an inspiration.

Donna Glasky, our book administrative assistant, was the glue that kept this project on time and on task when the editors were at risk of losing focus.

Donna's unending "can do" attitude and attention to detail supported us to assure that we kept our partnership for result.

Finally, PKL would like to acknowledge Mike Grisham for providing "the space" to create what we did at NeuroCare, and Joe Friedman for his contributing coaching, mentoring, and love.

Part I

Outcome-Based Clinical Rehabilitation

The purpose of Part I is to define outcome-oriented rehabilitation within the context of medical rehabilitation in America and to present principles for achievement of target results along the rehabilitation continuum.

Chapter 1

Rehab 2000: The Evolution of Medical Rehabilitation in American Health Care

Gerben DeJong, PhD, and Janet P. Sutton, PhD

Objectives

- To evaluate medical rehabilitation's growing role in American health care.
- To examine the major shifts in American health care that are likely to affect medical rehabilitation as we approach the year 2000.
- To examine recent trends in medical rehabilitation including the proliferation of rehabilitation facilities and the diversification of rehabilitation services.
- To present the thesis that payer-induced growth in medical rehabilitation reflects a larger shift in American health care from a provider-driven to a payer-driven system and that American health care will make yet another major shift to a more consumer-driven health care system in the future.
- To identify six key conditions or markers of a consumer-driven system and present implications of these for outcomes management and for purchasing of medical rehabilitation services in the future.

Medical rehabilitation is a $15 to $20 billion a year industry and is expected by some to exceed $45 billion by the year 2000.[1, 2] During the 1980s, medical rehabilitation emerged from relative obscurity to become an essential component of any health care network or system that claimed to provide the full continuum of care for those with major

The production of this chapter was supported in part by the NRH Research Center's Research & Training Center on Medical Rehabilitation Services & Health Policy (RTC-MRS&HP) which is funded with a grant from the National Institute on Disability & Rehabilitation Research (NIDRR). (Grant #H133B40025.) The views expressed in this chapter are those of the authors and do not necessarily reflect the views of the NRH Research Center, the National Rehabilitation Hospital, the Medlantic Research Institute, nor any other organization with which the authors are affiliated.

physical or cognitive impairments resulting from catastrophic injuries and chronic health conditions. Today, any health system that touts its sophisticated capacities for saving lives simply is no longer credible if it does not also provide an array of restorative services that enhance the residual functional capacities of patients with severe physical impairments. This newfound acceptance of medical rehabilitation as an essential health system component is one of the factors that have contributed to the rapid growth of the medical rehabilitation industry during the 1980s and early 1990s.

As the industry grows and matures, it is also changing. It serves a more diverse group of patients in more diverse settings. Medical rehabilitation has broadened its patient base from its original focus on groups such as those with polio, spinal cord injury, and stroke to a larger array of groups that also includes, for example, people with traumatic brain injury, long-term polio, and chronic work-related maladies such as low-back problems and repetitive motion disorders. Historically a hospital-based service program, medical rehabilitation today is also provided in a variety of outpatient settings, in skilled nursing facilities, and in the home. Some of these changes have been induced by the growth of managed health care plans that seek low cost alternatives to hospital-based care for all types of medical services.

PURPOSE AND SCOPE

This chapter seeks to discern where medical rehabilitation will be in the years ahead, especially as we turn the page from one century to the next in the year 2000. Before looking ahead, we want to glance backward to examine what has happened to the medical rehabilitation market over the last couple of decades. We take a market approach by first looking at the *demand side* of the market, then the *supply side*; the *role of fiscal intermediaries*; and finally the trend toward *corporatization and consolidation*.

While a market analysis of medical rehabilitation can help us discern and understand some of the trends in medical rehabilitation, it overlooks a fundamental shift in American health care that will impact the future of medical rehabilitation. *It is our thesis that American health care is currently moving from a provider- to a payer-driven system and will eventually move to a consumer-driven system. The payer-driven health care system that is now gaining momentum is only part of an extended transition to a more consumer-driven, risk-neutral, market-based health care system.* Future observers of American health policy will note that the real intent of comprehensive health care reform was to accelerate the transition to a more consumer-driven system. As we will note later, one of the underpinnings of a consumer-driven health care system will be the provision of services that are truly outcome-oriented. For medical rehabilitation to compete successfully in a consumer-driven health care system, it too will have to make outcomes a central feature in the delivery of its services.

WHAT IS MEDICAL REHABILITATION?

Medical rehabilitation seeks to enhance the residual functional abilities of people who have acquired a disabling impairment because of a congenital limitation, trauma, acute illness, chronic health condition, or other medical episode that has limited their ability to function independently. Medical rehabilitation's goal is to enable individuals to "live in the least restrictive, least costly environment at their highest possible level of independence."[3]

Medical rehabilitation includes a multidisciplinary array of evaluative, diagnostic, and therapeutic services rendered by physiatrists (physicians specializing in rehabilitation medicine), physical therapists, occupational therapists, speech and language therapists, nurses, prosthetists, orthotists, psychologists, social workers, vocational counselors, recreation therapists, and assistive technologists. One of medical rehabilitation's trademarks has been its strong commitment to an interdisciplinary team approach that attempts to address the full scope of patients' physical, emotional, and other support needs.[4]

According to 1992 data from the Uniform Data System for Medical Rehabilitation (UDS$_{MR}$), a national database to which over 700 hospital-based rehabilitation facilities currently contribute data, 64 percent of rehabilitation discharges are people with stroke and orthopedically related conditions such as hip fracture.[5] Other groups include people with spinal cord injuries, brain injuries, amputations, major multiple trauma, arthritis, congenital conditions, other neurological conditions, and burns. Medical rehabilitation also serves people with less severe impairments who have functional limitations resulting from minor injuries or from prolonged inactivity caused by an illness.

Medical rehabilitation services are provided in a variety of inpatient and outpatient settings. These include free-standing rehabilitation hospitals, rehabilitation units within acute care hospitals, hospital-based outpatient facilities, nonhospital comprehensive outpatient rehabilitation facilities (CORFs), "subacute" rehabilitation usually provided in skilled nursing facilities (SNFs), and home-based rehabilitation.

Although medical rehabilitation has been a feature of the American medical landscape for many years, it did not come into its own until World War II when returning veterans and survivors of the polio epidemics in the 1940s and 1950s created new populations who needed restorative care.[6] Over the years, medical rehabilitation has become more organized and has come to serve a broader group of people in a greater variety of settings.

Until recently, physiatrists, or physician specialists in medical rehabilitation, did not enjoy the same level of professional acceptance and legitimacy as did physicians practicing acute care medicine. This has changed as the rest of health care has awakened to the chronic nature and long-term functional consequences of many health conditions under the purview of other medical disciplines. Today medical rehabilitation is one of the fastest growing medical specialties, is able to attract well-qualified residents, and enjoys growing acceptance in academic medicine.

DEMAND AND SUPPLY

Demand

Nationwide, over 35 million individuals, or one-seventh of the population, have a health condition that limits one or more life activities.[7] The prevalence of chronic and disabling conditions is known to increase with age.[8] As noted in Table 1–1, 37.5 percent of persons aged 65 years and older have an activity limitation due to the presence of a chronic health condition; 10.6 percent are unable to carry on their major activity.* The percentage of individuals in each age group reporting activity limitations continues to show an upward trend (Table 1–1).[9]

---

*The National Center for Health Statistics (NCHS) defines an activity limitation as a "long-term reduction in a person's capacity to perform the usual kind or amount of activities associated with his or her age group." NCHS defines a major activity limitation as a limitation in a principal activity appropriate for an individual's age and gender, such as playing with children for individuals between the ages of 1 and 5 years, attending school for individuals between the ages of 5 and 17 years, and attending work or school for adults over the age of 18.

Table 1–1

Activity Limitations Caused by Chronic Health Conditions by Age: United States, 1987 and 1992*

Age	Total with Limitation of Activity		Limited but Not in Major Activity		Limited in Amount or Kind of Major Activity		Unable To Carry on Major Activity	
	1987	1992	1987	1992	1987	1992	1987	1992
	Percent of population							
All ages (total)	12.9	14.2	4.0	4.3	5.2	5.5	3.7	4.3
Age								
Under 15 years	4.7	5.8	1.3	1.5	3.0	3.8	0.4	0.6
15–44 years	8.1	9.9	2.6	3.0	3.4	4.0	2.0	2.9
45–64 years	22.3	22.8	5.6	5.6	8.2	7.8	8.5	9.3
65 years and over	37.5	38.8	14.7	15.6	12.9	12.5	10.0	10.6
65–74 years	34.7	34.4	12.8	13.6	11.3	10.4	10.7	10.4
75 years and over	41.9	45.3	17.7	18.6	15.4	15.7	8.9	11.1

*Note: Data are based on household interviews of a sample of the civilian noninstitutionalized population.

Source: Adapted from Centers for Disease Control and Prevention, National Center for Health Statistics, Division of Health Interview Statistics: Data from the National Health Interview Survey.

The demand for medical rehabilitation services will continue to increase as the population ages and as the number of people with functional limitations continues to increase. The elderly population constitutes the fastest growing segment of the U.S. population. Between 1980 and 1991, while the overall U.S. population increased by 11 percent, the population 65 years and over increased by 24 percent and the population 85 years and over increased by 41 percent. The ranks of the 65-and-older population will increase dramatically when the leading edge of the baby boom generation reaches retirement age in another 16 years.

Exogenous demographic trends alone do not adequately explain current or future demand for medical rehabilitation. Part of the increasing demand for medical rehabilitation is endogenous to the health care system, which has become extraordinarily successful in saving and extending lives, albeit often with a long-term impairment or functional limitation. As the mortality rate for many conditions continues to decline there often is a corresponding increase in disability.[10-12] Mortality and morbidity/disability rates are inversely related. Two examples are worth noting.

First, consider people with stroke, the largest impairment group served by medical rehabilitation. Each year over 500,000 Americans experience a stroke. Mortality from stroke, the third leading cause of death in the United States, declined 70 percent between 1970 and 1991 (see Figure 1–1). However, as the stroke mortality rate has declined, the number of survivors experiencing functional limitations has increased.

Deaths per 100,000 population

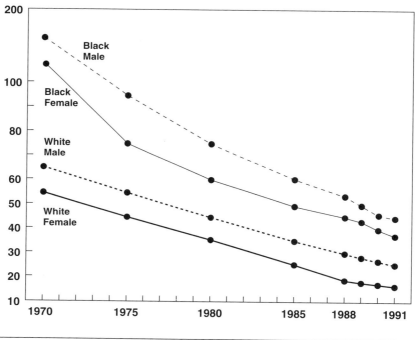

Race and sex	1970	1975	1980	1985	1988	1989	1990	1991
White male	68.8	56.7	41.9	33.0	30.3	28.4	27.7	26.9
Black male	122.5	95.0	77.5	62.7	60.8	57.3	56.1	54.9
White female	56.2	46.1	35.2	27.9	25.5	24.2	23.8	22.8
Black female	107.9	78.6	61.7	50.6	47.1	45.5	42.7	41.0

Figure 1–1 Stroke Mortality: Death Rates for Stroke by Race and Sex: United States, 1970–91

And, **second**, consider people with spinal cord injuries (SCIs) and traumatic brain injuries (TBIs), many of which result from motor vehicle crashes and falls. Between 1970 and 1991, mortality from motor vehicle accidents and falls declined 27 percent (Figure 1–2). This decline can be attributed, in part, to the advances made in emergency medicine systems, which are saving lives but often with significant impairments among new survivors.[†‡] One result has been an increase in the proportion of SCI survivors with quadriplegia and those with very high-level quadriplegia requiring some form of mechanical ventilation. Similarly, people with TBI are also better served by emergency medical systems. Prior to 1980,

Deaths per 100,000 population

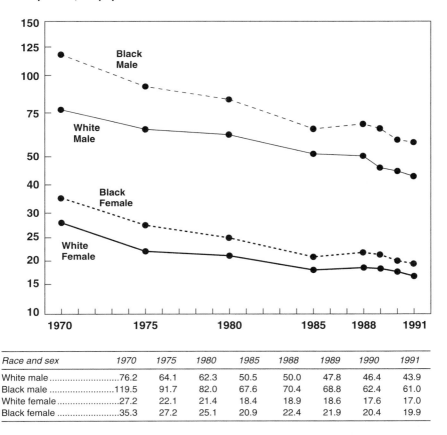

Race and sex	1970	1975	1980	1985	1988	1989	1990	1991
White male	76.2	64.1	62.3	50.5	50.0	47.8	46.4	43.9
Black male	119.5	91.7	82.0	67.6	70.4	68.8	62.4	61.0
White female	27.2	22.1	21.4	18.4	18.9	18.6	17.6	17.0
Black female	35.3	27.2	25.1	20.9	22.4	21.9	20.4	19.9

Figure 1–2 Unintentional Injury Mortality: Death Rates for Unintentional Injuries by Race and Sex: United States, 1970–91

[†]Improved emergency medical systems may also help to reduce the degree of morbidity and disability among groups who previously were not predicted to survive. For example, in spinal cord injury, there has been an increase in the number of incomplete injuries. In recent years, new clinical protocols call for massive doses of methylprednisolone in the first few hours following an injury. Such interventions are intended to prevent secondary injuries due to swelling and thereby reduce the extent of secondary disability.

[‡]This decline can also be attributed, in part, to improvements in the crash-worthiness of motor vehicles.

organized TBI rehabilitation services were virtually nonexistent. Today, people with TBI comprise 4 percent of all persons discharged from hospital-based rehabilitation programs.[5]

Changes in the demographic and epidemiologic characteristics of disability provide some indication of how the overall need/demand for medical rehabilitation is changing over time. However, the data presented previously do not provide adequate impairment-specific information on the need and demand for medical rehabilitation. Methods for making demand and bed-need estimates for medical rehabilitation in specific markets remain crude, and published national demand estimates do not currently exist.[§]

Supply

Hospital-Based Rehabilitation

Traditionally, medical rehabilitation services have been provided in inpatient settings within either free-standing rehabilitation hospitals or rehabilitation units of acute care hospitals. From 1985 to 1994, the number of free-standing rehabilitation hospitals increased 175 percent from 68 to 187 hospitals (Table 1–2). During this same period, the number of rehabilitation units increased by 118 percent, from 386 to 804 units.[2]

Medical rehabilitation services are also provided in facilities classified as long-term care hospitals, a diverse collection of hospitals that serve many of the same patient populations served in traditional rehabilitation hospitals and units. These hospitals also serve patients with a variety of chronic and terminal conditions who are not candidates for organized rehabilitation services. From 1985 to 1994, the number of long-term hospitals increased by 31 percent, from 86 to 113 hospitals (Table 1–2).

Alternatives to Hospital-Based Rehabilitation

Despite the proliferation of hospitals and units providing rehabilitative care, the growth rate in the number of hospital-based rehabilitation facilities is declining as alternative sources of rehabilitation such as skilled nursing facilities (SNFs)—often referred to as subacute care facilities—and outpatient facilities expand.

[§]The Research and Training Center in Medical Rehabilitation Services and Health Policy (RTC-MRS&HP), a division of the National Rehabilitation Hospital Research Center in Washington, DC, is currently exploring the use of hospital discharge survey data as a means for developing demand estimates for medical rehabilitation.

Table 1–2

Yearly Estimates of the Number of Rehabilitation Facilities, SNFs, and
Long-Term Care Hospitals in the United States: 1985–1994

Type of Facility	1985	1987	1989	1991	1993	1994[6]	Percent Change 1985– 1994
Rehabilitation Hospitals[1]	68	88	125	152	180	187	+175
Rehabilitation Units[2]	386	539	642	672	783	804	+118
Long-term Care Hospitals[3]	86	87	89	91	109	113	+31
Skilled Nursing Facilities (SNFs)[4]	6,725	7,379	8,688	10,061	11,309	11,436	+70
Comprehensive Outpatient Rehabilitation Facilities (CORFs)[5]	86	141	184	201	229	237	+176

[1]Number of hospitals excluded from coverage under the Medicare PPS.
[2]Number of units excluded from coverage under the Medicare PPS.
[3]Number of long-term care hospitals excluded from coverage under the Medicare PPS.
[4]Number of SNFs participating in Medicare.
[5]Number of CORFs participating in Medicare.
[6]As of August 1994.

Source: Reprinted from *Trends in Medical Rehabilitation* by S. Wolk and T. Blair with permission of the American Rehabilitation Association, ©1994.

Skilled nursing facilities (SNFs). Skilled nursing facilities vary considerably in the mix and intensity of the rehabilitation services they provide, making it difficult to generalize about the character of rehabilitation services provided within the subacute portion of the industry. Nonetheless, the number of SNFs has increased considerably. From 1985 to 1994, the number increased 70 percent from 6,725 to 11,436 facilities[2] (Table 1–2).¶ Skilled nursing facilities probably represent the fastest growing part of the rehabilitation industry today.

Comprehensive Outpatient Rehabilitation Facilities (CORFs). As their name suggests, CORFs provide a fairly comprehensive array of medical rehabilitation services including vigorous day treatment programs for those whose medical and nursing needs do not require 24-hour inpatient supervision or management. From 1985 to 1994, the number of CORFs increased 176 percent from 86 to 237 (Table 1–2).¶

Other Outpatient Rehabilitation. Other outpatient rehabilitation facilities range from hospital-based outpatient programs to hospital-based satellite outpatient centers to free-standing outpatient centers.

¶On the basis of data from the Prospective Payment Advisory Commission[13], there were 580,929 Medicare or Medicaid certified skilled nursing beds in 1991.

Rehabilitation in a hospital-based outpatient setting is frequently provided after an acute stay, when patients have only minor limitations in functioning or when health insurance does not cover inpatient rehabilitation.[14] Between 1979 and 1990, the number of hospitals in the United States with an organized outpatient department increased from 35 percent to 85 percent. During this same period, the number of community hospitals having an organized outpatient rehabilitation program increased from 18 percent to 52 percent.[13]

Home-Based Rehabilitation. Among the newer entrants into the rehabilitation field are providers of comprehensive home-based rehabilitation services. The exact size of this portion of the industry is unknown. However, less organized in-home rehabilitation in the form of physical and occupational therapy has been a long-standing service provided by home health agencies, another fast-growing segment of American health care. In 1993, there were over 11,000 home health providers, 15 percent more than in the previous year. In a 1989 study of postacute care for Medicare patients, Neu and colleagues found that 27 percent of stroke patients received homecare after discharge.[15] Over one-third of patients discharged from acute care after a major joint, hip, or femur procedure also received home health services.

Total Supply

The total supply of rehabilitation services is difficult to gauge because rehabilitation services can range from highly organized comprehensive inpatient services to intermittent delivery of physical and occupational therapy in a variety of outpatient settings including the home. In recent years the growth of the inpatient rehabilitation capacity has tapered off while the growth of SNF-based and outpatient-based rehabilitation has accelerated.

Utilization and Costs

From 1986 to 1992, occupancy rates in rehabilitation hospitals and units fluctuated within a fairly narrow band from 68.1 percent to 76.6 percent (Table 1–3).[2] Utilization relative to supply or capacity on the outpatient side of the industry is difficult to gauge since there is no benchmark, such as the number of beds.

The average length of stay in rehabilitation hospitals and units decreased 14.3 percent in just 3 years from 28 days in 1990 to 24 days in 1992.[5]

Between 1986 and 1992, average per diem operating costs for Medicare patients increased from $330 to $567 for free-standing hospitals and from $381 to $576 for units (Table 1–3). Thus, despite declining average length of stay during this period, the average cost per discharge increased from $8,383 to $13,010 for free-standing hospitals and from $8,706 to $10,916 for units (Table 1–3).

Table 1–3

Occupancy Rates, Length of Stay, Cost per Diem and Costs per Discharge*: In-patient Medical Rehabilitation 1986–1992

Year	Occupancy Rates (%)		Avg. Length of Stay (days)		Cost per Diem ($)		Cost per Discharge ($)	
	Hospitals	Units	Hospital	Units	Hospital	Units	Hospital	Units
1986	76.6	72.1	28.9	25.9	$330	$381	$8,383	$8,706
1987	68.1	71.8	29.0	26.5	369	405	8,613	9,053
1988	69.5	71.8	28.5	24.4	415	436	10,175	9,397
1989	69.0	72.2	29.7	24.0	441	465	10,877	9,958
1990	72.0	71.1	27.6	22.9	480	497	12,743	10,625
1991	75.6	71.7	26.4	22.0	537	540	12,890	10,738
1992	73.3	70.3	25.6	21.1	567	576	13,010	10,916

Note: Numbers such as "cost per diem" may be understated since our data sources may have excluded certain outliers (e.g., facilities with costs one standard deviation above the mean). For this reason, the cost-per-diem and cost-per-discharge figures appear very low.

Source: Reprinted from *Trends in Medical Rehabilitation* by S. Wolk and T. Blair with permission of the American Rehabilitation Association, ©1994. Data from the Health Care Financing Administration, Minimum Data Sets, Baltimore, Maryland.

*Medicare only.

Although the average length of stay is decreasing, average functional gain per day or per week of inpatient rehabilitation, as gauged by the functional independence measure (FIM), is increasing.† In other words, inpatient rehabilitation providers are accomplishing more for each hospital day.[5]

Role of Fiscal Intermediaries

The rapid growth of the medical rehabilitation industry cannot be explained solely by increasing demand. One could argue that the growth

---

†Gain in functioning per day is also referred to as length-of-stay (LOS) efficiency.

in the supply of medical rehabilitation is merely a response to unmet need and that the industry is simply catching up. However, medical rehabilitation has never been a demand- or consumer-driven industry. Like that of many other health services, the delivery of medical rehabilitation services has been shaped by powerful incentives inherent in the policies of fiscal intermediaries wedged between the demand and supply sides of the market.[16]

Payers of Medical Rehabilitation

Despite the size of the medical rehabilitation industry, remarkably scant information is available on the extent to which public and private payers provide coverage for medical rehabilitation. In terms of 1988–1990 data from UDS$_{MR}$, 70 percent of individuals admitted to a rehabilitation hospital or distinct part unit are covered by Medicare; 21 percent are covered by private payers such as Blue Cross, health maintenance organizations (HMOs), and other commercial insurers; 4 percent are covered by Medicaid; and the remaining 4 percent are covered by workers' compensation, CHAMPUS, federal-state vocational rehabilitation (VR) programs, and self-pay (Table 1–4). Clearly, the federal government, through the Medicare, Medicaid, CHAMPUS, and VR programs, is the principal payer of inpatient medical rehabilitation services. The national payer mix for medical rehabilitation in nonhospital settings remains largely unknown.

Table 1–4

Primary Payment Source 1988–90: In-patient Medical Rehabilitation

Payer	Percent
Medicare	70.1
Commercial Insurance	19.0
Worker's Compensation/Other	4.6
Medicaid	4.2
HMO	2.1
Total	100.00

N=79,996.

Source: Data from the Uniform Data System for Medical Rehabilitation, 1990.

Medicare. As the single largest payer of medical rehabilitation services, Medicare has been a major force in shaping the delivery and availability of medical rehabilitation services. Medicare Part A covers inpatient rehabilitation provided by rehabilitation hospitals and units; Part B covers outpatient rehabilitation services rendered in various types of outpatient centers including comprehensive outpatient rehabilitation facilities (CORFs). Medicare Parts A and B cover rehabilitation services in the home when rendered as part of a specific episode of care.

Despite the scope of Medicare coverage, medical rehabilitation services account for only 1.5 percent of all Medicare expenditures.[16]* Nonetheless, inpatient medical rehabilitation continues to be a fast-growing segment within the Medicare program. Between 1989 and 1991, inpatient rehabilitation facilities experienced a 42 percent increase in the number of Medicare cases, from 144,252 to 204,213.[17]

Medicaid. Rehabilitation services are also covered under the federal-state Medicaid program, which is mainly available to participants in the Aid to Families with Dependent Children (AFDC) program and the Supplemental Security Income (SSI) program, including people who qualify because of a disability.** Because of the discretion allowed to each state, Medicaid benefits and policies vary across states. Although Medicaid remains the single largest payer of nursing home care in the United States,[18] the extent to which it is a payer of SNF-based rehabilitation is unknown.††

Private Plans. The majority of individuals in the United States are insured through private health plans. Private health insurance coverage for medical rehabilitation varies greatly and the full extent of private coverage for medical rehabilitation remains largely unknown. Traditional indemnity plans such as those marketed by Blue Cross and Blue Shield generally provide good coverage for inpatient medical rehabilitation. However, managed care plans, in the form of HMOs, preferred provider organizations (PPOs), and other arrangements, are rapidly displacing tra-

---

*We strongly suspect that Medicare also pays for many other rehabilitationlike services that may never be billed as medical rehabilitation services.

**People who would otherwise qualify for AFDC and SSI, but whose income and resources are too high, may still qualify for Medicaid if their income and resources do not exceed state-determined income and resource standards. These individuals, while not "categorically eligible," are deemed "categorically related."

††Medicaid reimbursement is often quite meager compared to that of other payer sources. It is doubtful that Medicaid is a major source of payment for the rapidly expanding SNF portion of the rehabilitation industry.

ditional indemnity plans in many health care markets in the nation.[‡,§,¶] Managed care plans have typically not provided coverage for rehabilitation beyond the minimum benefit package required for federal qualification. Indeed, the number of HMOs contracting with rehabilitation centers continues to be small.[19]

Payment Policy and the Impact of Managed Care

PPS exemption and TEFRA limits. In 1983, payment of acute hospital care shifted from a retrospective payment system based on cost to a prospective payment system (PPS) based on diagnosis related groups (DRGs). When Congress enacted PL 98-21, the statutory basis for DRGs, it exempted medical rehabilitation in the belief that the DRG classification system was suitable for acute care but not for rehabilitation.[13,22–24] Instead, Medicare payment for medical rehabilitation would continue to be cost-based, subject to certain limits established under the Tax Equity and Fiscal Responsibility Act (TEFRA) of 1982.

The PPS exemption for medical rehabilitation created powerful incentives for acute care hospital providers to develop new inpatient rehabilitation programs, in part to accommodate patients with costs that were expected to exceed DRG payment limits. As noted earlier, medical rehabilitation began its rapid growth in the mid-1980s.

Medical care inflation continues to outpace the annual increases in TEFRA target limits for rehabilitation facilities. Approximately half of all PPS-exempt rehabilitation facilities have costs that equal or exceed their TEFRA limits, a phenomenon that may account for the significant reduction in length of stay cited earlier. Moreover, there is mounting concern that serious inequities exist in the determination of hospital costs and that many rehabilitation facilities are exposed to additional financial risk because of differences in casemix or patient severity.

These concerns have fueled interest in the development of a prospective payment for inpatient rehabilitation facilities. Currently, significant efforts are being devoted to the development of patient classification and payment models that address these inequities in TEFRA reimbursement.

---

‡In 1993, HMOs alone covered 19.4 percent of the U.S. population. Massachusetts, at 38.9 percent of the population, and California, at 36.4 percent of the population, had the highest levels of HMO penetration.[19]

§Even the Blues are converting their plans to the managed care variety. "Currently about 42 percent of the Blues plans' total enrollment—27.3 million out of 65.5 million—is in managed care."[20]

¶In 1993, more than half (53 percent) of all persons enrolled in employer-sponsored health plans participated in a managed care plan.[21] This figure is expected to increase to 90 percent by the year 2000.

Since the focus of inpatient rehabilitation is patient function, a payment system that focuses on functional status is generating substantial interest among policymakers and rehabilitation specialists.[13, 25-27]

Impact of Managed Care. Among private payers, indemnity-based health plans such as Blue Cross and Blue Shield plans have reimbursed rehabilitation providers retrospectively on the basis of charges or costs. This source of private sector payment, as noted earlier, is becoming less important as managed care plans have displaced traditional indemnity plans. While it is difficult to generalize about the nature of managed care contracts with rehabilitation providers, managed care plans typically channel patients to "network" providers such as hospitals that have agreed to accept a predetermined or heavily discounted price.

More significant for medical rehabilitation is the extent to which the Medicare program, inpatient rehabilitation's largest payer, is rapidly shifting toward the use of managed care contracts in many markets. In 1993, only 5 percent of Medicare beneficiaries were enrolled in managed care plans nationwide.[¶] Anecdotal evidence suggests that the percentage is increasing very rapidly.

The growth of managed care is having a major effect on the rehabilitation industry's provider mix and is driving the rapid shift to nonhospital rehabilitation alternatives such as SNF-based subacute rehabilitation and outpatient rehabilitation. The American Rehabilitation Association (AmRehab) believes that the rapid growth of subacute care can also be attributed to other payer-induced behaviors. AmRehab cites, for instance, how acute care hospitals have developed subacute beds "to get DRG outliers out of acute beds" and how Medicare's 3-hour therapy rule for inpatient medical rehabilitation may have spurred the development of subacute care for patients who cannot benefit from 3 hours of therapy per day.[2]

Corporatization and Consolidation of Rehabilitation

The 1980s and the first half of the 1990s have witnessed unprecedented growth in the number of mergers and acquisitions in American health care. In 1992, 43 percent of all hospitals were organized as part of a multihospital system, compared to 28 percent in 1980.[29] The mergers-and-acquisitions fever has also spread to inpatient medical rehabilitation.

[¶]In certain markets, the proportion of Medicare beneficiaries enrolled in HMOs is substantially higher. For example, 20 percent of beneficiaries in California and 22 percent in Arizona are enrolled in HMOs.[28]

In its 1991 hospital survey, the American Hospital Association[30] found that approximately 37 percent of rehabilitation hospitals and 51 percent of units were organized as part of a multihospital system.

Similar trends can be found in the nursing home industry. Between 1992 and 1993, 14 of the largest 32 nursing home chains increased their number of facilities. During this same period four new home health chains appeared.[31]

Four main trends in the organization of medical rehabilitation can be discerned. First is *diversification,* the trend among established rehabilitation providers to offer a larger array of services in a greater variety of settings ranging from hospitals to satellite outpatient centers. This trend can be attributed to Medicare and managed care payment policies (as previously described, e.g., TEFRA limits) that have led providers to develop less costly out-of-hospital alternatives.

Second is *vertical integration,* the trend of rehabilitation providers to become vertically integrated with a larger network of health care providers within a given health care market. This trend can be attributed to the desire of rehabilitation providers to have a steady stream of patients from acute care to rehabilitative care. Moreover, vertically integrated provider networks are in a better position to negotiate with health plans in providing a continuum of health services. Of the four trends, this trend is perhaps the most well established.

Third is *horizontal integration,* the trend of rehabilitation providers to become a horizontally integrated part of a national multihospital or multiprovider chain providing similar services across markets. This trend can be attributed to the desire of rehabilitation providers to achieve economies of scale and thus reduce costs in a more price-competitive health care economy.

And fourth is *within market consolidation,* the trend of established rehabilitation providers to consolidate, merge, or forge ad hoc partnerships with existing or potential competitors within markets that are already saturated with similar rehabilitation providers. This trend can be attributed to the excess capacity that results when there are too many existing or potentially similar providers in a given market.[##]

[##]These trends are not easily discerned, in part, because there is not a large trade-based literature that tracks these kinds of trends. The first periodical to monitor some of these trends is the recently introduced *Rehab Management,* a publication aimed at the business side of medical rehabilitation. These days, one can sometimes learn more about the medical rehabilitation industry by reading the *Wall Street Journal* than by keeping up with the industry's professional journals except, perhaps, for the journals' recruitment ads that provide some indication as to where new providers are emerging.

The third trend, horizontal integration, especially the growth of national multihospital chains, is not easily explained for three reasons. First, payer demand in the market is for lower-level or subacute care, not for traditional inpatient care. Second, the economies of scale that are often claimed for multihospital chains have intrinsic limits. As national multihospital chains become larger, they eventually become burdened with new corporate overhead at either the regional or the national level or both. The economies of scale in purchasing materials and supplies can also be achieved through better vertical integration with other health care facilities in the same market. And third, most health care markets are essentially regional, not national, in character. The market strength of a rehabilitation provider is its ability to position itself regionally, not nationally.

Multihospital chains are, however, in a better position to raise large amounts of capital through stock offerings or from venture capital, a capacity that is often well beyond the scope of smaller free-standing or regionally based rehabilitation systems. Smaller not-for-profit systems are limited to raising capital by increasing their debt load, thereby adding to their cost structure and reducing their ability to be price competitive. The growth of multihospital chains is driven more by the nature of capital markets and the price demands of managed care plans than by the fundamentals of supply and demand within regional markets.

In the present health care environment there exists great uncertainty about the future of health care and health care reform. Integrated organizations are perhaps better positioned to adapt to this uncertain market. Larger organized systems will possess greater bargaining power than smaller unorganized systems if consumer purchasing alliances are included as part of a health care reform effort. Vertically integrated organizations, for example, are more capable of providing services throughout the continuum of care[32] and thus are more attractive to potential payers. In the face of this uncertainty, health care analysts expect that future growth in medical rehabilitation will derive largely from joint ventures or other types of partnerships between providers.[33]

TOWARD A CONSUMER-DRIVEN HEALTH CARE SYSTEM

The hospital-based portion of the medical rehabilitation industry has, it is safe to say, been blindsided by the growth of managed care and the rapid development of non–hospital-based alternatives. This portion of the industry was immune to larger managed care trends mainly because of its dependence on Medicare, which, until recently, remained a cost-based and a fee-for-service payment system.

Medical rehabilitation's current preoccupation with managed care, however, will be misplaced if it does not also consider the larger shifts in American health care noted in the opening sections of this paper: that is, the shift from a provider- to a payer-driven health care system now under way and the shift from a payer- to a consumer-driven system soon to emerge.

The distinctions among provider-, payer-, and consumer-driven health care systems are noteworthy, and their differences can provide considerable insight as to the future direction of American health care and medical rehabilitation's role in it. The differing provider, payer, and consumer systems constitute the analytic framework for the balance of this chapter and are outlined in Table 1–5. We will argue that medical rehabilitation needs to brace itself for the consumer-driven health care system that will inevitably come, the outlines of which are readily apparent in many of the health care reform proposals that surfaced in the 103 Congress (1993–94). Finally, we will argue that medical rehabilitation, because of its long-standing attention to outcome measurement and database development, will have many, but not all of the important tools needed to compete successfully in a more consumer-driven health care system.

Provider-Driven Health Care

Historically, American health care has been a provider-driven, if not a provider-controlled system. Paternalism and physician-knows-best attitudes were at one time prominent features of American health care. Because of providers' advanced training and claim to scientific legitimacy, their opinions often went unchallenged. Credentialing, certification, and accreditation were surrogates for quality. There was a heavy emphasis on the input side of the production function as reflected in the accreditation criteria used by the Joint Commission on the Accreditation of Healthcare Organizations (JCAHO), which provided hospitals the "Good Housekeeping Seal of Approval." There was little emphasis on the output side apart from the elimination of pathologic conditions and the

Table 1–5

Chapter's Analytic Framework
Comparing Provider-, Payer-, Consumer-Driven Health Care Systems

Dimension	Provider- Driven (Supply Side)	Payer-Driven (Intermediary)	Consumer-Driven (Demand Side)
Key value	Provider autonomy	Cost minimization	Consumer sovereignty
Basis of competition	Prestige and risk	Price and risk	Price and quality
Economic goals	Revenue maximization	Market share/ profit maximization	Cost-effectiveness (efficiency)
Pricing	"Usual and customary"	Discounting	Value-based
Method of payment	Fee-for-service	Case mix (eg, DRGs, FRGs), RBRVS capitation	Risk-adjusted capitation, carve-outs
Quality	Accreditation Credentialing	Perception of quality, CQI, TQM	Outcomes, consumer satisfaction
Access	Provider-controlled	Payer-controlled	Consumer choice
Capacity	Excess capacity	Reduced capacity	Balanced capacity
Utilization	Overutilization	Underservice	Balanced
Utilization review	Retrospective	Prospective	Not needed
Costs	Not important	Very important	Relative to outcome
Outcomes	Elimination of pathology, "satisficing"	Reduced utilization reduced costs	Health status, functional status, quality of life, consumer satisfaction
Outcome disclosure	Confidential/secret	Selective disclosure	Full disclosure
Providers as price takers	No	Yes	Yes
Homogeneous product	No	No	Yes, standard benefit package
Knowledge and expertise	Rests with provider	Second-guessed by payer	Made accessible to consumer
Rating	Experience rating	Experience rating	Community rating
Risk adjustment	No	Some case-mix adjustment	Yes
Governance	Provider-dominated	Payer-dominated	Consumer-dominated

reduction of mortality. Outcomes related to functional ability and quality of life were thought to be conceptually too fuzzy, immeasurable, and beyond the legitimate domain of acute care medicine.

Provider autonomy, both clinical autonomy and regulatory autonomy, is the most cherished value in a provider-driven system.[34] Provider autonomy also means controlling resources and choosing which patients providers are willing to accept. In exchange for this autonomy, providers are expected to act as agents in promoting their patients' best interests. The provider's fiduciary responsibility is to the patient, not to the payer.

Competition in a provider-driven system is based on prestige, not on price and quality (except for the structural indicators of quality commonly surveyed by accrediting bodies). Thus, providers compete on the basis of the latest technology, their academic affiliations, the credentials and size of their medical staff, their level of specialization, and the bed size of their institutions. Although prestige-based competition has helped to make American health care the most sophisticated and technologically advanced in the world, it has also led to tremendous excess capacity that has made it frightfully expensive and unaffordable for many.

American health care has defied the usual laws of supply and demand. In normal markets, excess supply results in lower prices; in health care, excess supply results in higher prices and overutilization. This can be attributed, in part, to the fee-for-service and cost-based methods of reimbursement, which enabled providers to determine what services should be provided, in what quantities, and at what prices. This deference to provider autonomy was also incorporated into the original Medicare legislation, which set physician fees based on charges deemed to be "usual and customary."

Payer-Driven Health Care

While providers honored their fiduciary responsibilities to their patients, there was never a corresponding social contract with society as a whole to create self-imposed constraints on provider appetites for technology, increased capacity, and revenue maximization. In the absence of a genuinely competitive market to discipline provider behavior, a whole host of payer-determined constraints have been imposed over the years such as utilization review, DRG payment for hospitals, and resource-based relative value scale (RBRVS) for physician payment. While these mechanisms limited provider autonomy, providers have learned to live with them or, in many instances, have tried to outgame these limits in pursuit of traditional provider-driven objectives such as revenue maximization.

The failure of these mechanisms to rein in health care costs fully has accelerated the development of managed care plans. Many larger employers find managed care plans to be an attractive way to hold down costs and keep the prices of their products and the salaries of their employees competitive.

Managed care plans challenge the autonomy that providers have heretofore enjoyed. Instead of *retrospective* utilization review, "case managers" representing managed care plans make *prospective* reviews as to whether the patient needs the care recommended. Horror stories abound about how physicians are being micromanaged, second-guessed, and financially penalized when their patient costs exceed predetermined targets. In a payer-driven system the ultimate financial control of patient care shifts from the provider to the payer.

Managed care plans seek to maximize market share through discounting. They attempt to maximize their financial gain by limiting expenditures and by marketing to lower-risk populations. Managed care plans create powerful incentives to underserve high-risk populations such as those typically served in rehabilitation settings.

Thus, managed care plans compete mainly on the basis of price and risk, not on quality or outcome despite the frequent lip service made to quality. Managed care plans nonetheless expect their provider network to be perceived as credible in order to market their plans to prospective subscriber groups successfully. Likewise, providers seeking managed care contracts will work hard to maintain the perception of quality, hence the popularity of continuous quality improvement (CQI) and total quality management (TQM). There cannot be, however, genuine competition on quality/outcome unless there is full disclosure of outcomes that also takes into account the case mix of individual providers or networks of providers. Outcome competition in the absence of independent verification and case-mix adjustment is virtually meaningless.

One exception to this observation is payers who have a long-term financial interest such as reinsurers and some workers' compensation firms who manage catastrophic injury cases. Reinsurers, for example, become involved when the medical and rehabilitation costs of an injury are likely to exceed a predetermined dollar threshold (e.g., $250,000). What makes reinsurance distinctive is that it has long-term financial liability and will attempt to allocate resources efficiently in order to avert downstream complications and costs.[***] Payers with long-term financial liability are also more open to performance-based or outcome-based contracting on a case-by-case basis.

[***]Payers whose financial liability does not extend beyond the person's current enrollment period have every incentive to make life difficult for the claimant in the hope that the case will become another payer's headache.

We believe that the combined weaknesses of both the provider- and payer-driven systems will eventually give way to a consumer-driven health care system where there will be genuine competition based on price and quality/outcome. We believe that medical rehabilitation will only thrive in an outcome-oriented level playing field created by a consumer-driven health care system.

Consumer-Driven Health Care

We predict that by the year 2000 the American health care system will have many of the elements of a consumer-driven system. We believe that the rules of the game will change gradually but dramatically and that we will begin to see meaningful competition based on price and quality where outcomes are a central feature in the purchase of health plans and the selection of medical rehabilitation providers. We believe that the movement toward a consumer-driven system is inexorable and unstoppable.

With the health care reform debate during the 103 Congress (1993–94) the nation made a major attempt to move toward a more consumer-driven health care system but faltered. We did not take the steps needed to implement a consumer-driven system, in part, because we had not yet completed the transition from a provider- to a payer-driven system, let alone a consumer-driven one. Because managed care plans were relatively new products in many markets, many people still did not have sufficient firsthand familiarity with the downside of managed care, although many had seen their choices in providers slip away. Moreover, a consumer-driven system represented a threat to those with a vested interest in the provider-driven and payer-driven systems. Finally, the proponents of a consumer-driven system failed to communicate to the public its essential components and how such a system would empower the purchasing decisions of the consumer.

We want to make clear that in speaking about a consumer-driven system we are speaking about consumers primarily as *informed purchasers* of health care services and secondarily as *informed users* of health care services such as medical rehabilitation. Consumers are learning how to become informed users of nonemergent health care services and some have even learned to second-guess their providers by tapping into the medical research literature to obtain information on the outcomes of alternative procedures, especially in the case of life-threatening health conditions. However, consumers remain woefully uninformed about how to choose a health plan or how to choose a provider, mainly because outcomes at the health-plan level and the provider level are either not available or not made accessible to consumers.

Six Conditions

There are six essential conditions or components of a consumer-driven health care system. The first three of these components are derived from the economic theory of "perfect competition," and the second three are idiosyncratic to the purchasing and provision of health care services. All six of these conditions can also be used as criteria by which to judge the adequacy of various health care reform proposals. All six of these conditions or components have major implications for the marketing of medical rehabilitation services and the development of outcome-based market competition in medical rehabilitation.

All these conditions are not likely to be fully attained. To the extent to which they are largely attained, we can say that we have a consumer-driven system. We expect that health care will, over the next several years, move vigorously in the direction of a consumer-directed system that will meet most, if not all, of the conditions outlined in the discussion that follows. Some of these conditions will be more fully implemented than others.

Conditions Derived from the Theory of Perfect Competition

1. Price takers: Health care plans and providers are price takers, not price makers. A key assumption in the theory of perfect competition is that **producers are price takers:** they do not set prices; prices are set by the market, based on what consumers collectively are willing to pay. If producers cannot sell a product at market price, they produce something else or go out of business. Historically, in health care, providers set prices as reflected in the Medicare policy of "usual and customary prices" noted earlier. Moreover, consumers are often in no position to negotiate the price, especially in an emergent situation. The time to negotiate price is before one becomes ill, injured, or impaired.[†††]

[†††]Once a person becomes ill, injured, or impaired, the price of health care services becomes very inelastic; people are willing to pay almost any price, even for marginally effective health care, in the hope of getting better. The price of health care is more elastic when people are healthy and examine the cost of a health plan against the probability that they will become ill, injured, or impaired and therefore will need large amounts of health care.

Managed care has turned the tables on providers by making them price takers rather than price makers. The problem, as noted earlier, is that the decision to include a provider in a managed care network is often driven largely by price and not by price *and quality.*

Almost every health care reform proposal presented in the 103 Congress sought to make both health plans and providers price takers by organizing consumers into large purchasing pools known as health insurance purchasing cooperatives (HIPCs) or health alliances.[‡‡‡] Whether "mandatory" or "voluntary," larger insurance pools will enhance consumer market power and bring greater price consciousness to the health care marketplace. One can begin to observe the emergence of voluntary purchasing pools in various markets and in various state-based health care reform plans.

2. Homogeneous product: Health care products are homogeneous: that is, health plans are organized around a standard benefit package. The concept of a **homogeneous product** is the second key assumption in the theory of perfect competition. There can be no effective price competition in the absence of a homogeneous product. In everyday commerce, we compare prices among similar goods. We can compare, for example, the price of Post raisin bran with that of Kellogg raisin bran. Moreover, we can compare the price and quality of roughly similar goods, for example, the price of a Honda Accord with that of a Mazda 626 or a Toyota Camry. Consumers cannot compare prices and quality unless they are comparing apples with apples and oranges with oranges.[§§§] Nor can they compare the price and quality of health plans unless they are comparing on the basis of a standard benefit package. Comparing competing health plans today, when a choice is still available, is almost impossible.[¶¶¶]

[‡‡‡]The principal difference between health care reform proposals in the 103 Congress was whether purchasing cooperatives or health alliances should be "mandatory" or "voluntary." This difference has major implications in terms of whether health plans can continue to compete on the basis of risk.

[§§§]When *Consumer Reports* compares the price, performance, and safety features of various automobiles in its articles, it almost always compares similar classes of automobiles. It does not, for example, make side-by-side comparisons of a Ford Escort with a Mercedes Benz. It compares automobiles in the same class.

[¶¶¶]A standardized benefit package is also important to creating a more risk-neutral playing field. By tweaking the composition of their benefit packages, health plans attempt to attract younger and healthier populations.

The principal challenge for medical rehabilitation is to have its services included in the standard benefit package around which health care plans compete. Rehabilitation providers will have to be able to (1) define their benefit packages in fairly generic terms (though they may be tailored to the needs of individual patients); (2) define expected outcomes, not only in rehabilitation and functional terms, but also in more generic terms at the health-plan level; and (3) set a price on the basis of which health plans can determine whether they will include the provider in its plan or network. Health plans also want to know about the capabilities and past performance of prospective providers.

In order to develop a level playing field for medical rehabilitation, the industry will have to develop a standardized way for providers to compete for health plan contracts. In the absence of an industry standard, health plans, health alliances, or government will define the terms of such competition.

3. Consumer knowledge: Consumers have ready access to information about prices and quality upon which to make informed decisions. **Perfect knowledge** is the third key assumption of perfect competition. While knowledge is never perfect, an informed consumer is essential to a consumer-driven and well-functioning competitive market. The problem with today's provider- and payer-driven health care systems is that there is little basis on which a consumer can make informed choices. First, when choosing health plans, the consumer has no basis on which to compare the quality of one plan with that of another. Second, when selecting providers within plans, the consumer again has little basis on which to compare one provider with another and often has to rely on the word-of-mouth recommendations made by friends and associates or on the perceptions created by the marketing departments of individual providers.

In the case of physicians, for example, past disciplinary action included in the National Practitioner Data Bank is not public information. The data bank is a federal repository containing information on malpractice payments, loss of licensure, or adverse actions taken against physicians, nurses, and other health professionals. This information is available to hospitals when determining whether to grant a physician admitting privileges but is not available to the public.[111]

In a consumer-driven health care system, consumer knowledge will be enhanced in two main ways. First will be the disclosure of standardized health-plan and provider outcomes that consumers will be able to use when selecting a health plan or a provider within a health plan. And second will be the use of consumer satisfaction ratings of individual health plans and individual providers within plans. These ratings will address issues such as satisfaction with the amenities provided, the courtesy of the provider staff, and the consumer's overall perception about the benefits obtained. Consumer ratings are already being used to a limited degree in some markets. For example, in the Washington, DC, area, *Consumer Checkbook,* the local analog to Consumers Union's *Consumer Reports,* provides a limited rating of health plans and individual provider ratings completed by its readers. In Wisconsin and Missouri, *Health Pages*, a consumer-oriented health publication, also seeks to rate health plans and health providers. *Health Pages* is expected to be in 11 other major health markets by the end of 1995.

Leading the way from a payer- to a consumer-driven health care system are larger employers who are demanding that health plans, especially managed care plans, provide standardized outcome and consumer satisfaction data. Large employers have market power that is akin to the purchasing power of health insurance purchasing cooperatives. As purchasers of managed care plans, large employers are leading the way in developing purchasing standards, supporting outcomes research, and conducting consumer satisfaction surveys. Large employers have contributed to the development of the Healthplan Employer Data and Information Set (HEDIS), which is beginning to provide high-quality data on managed care plans that can assist employers in making purchasing decisions. These initiatives, born out of the information needs of larger purchasers, will come to serve the needs of individual consumers in a more consumer-driven market since the information interests of large purchasers and small consumers are, in many ways, similar.

While the conditions for a consumer-driven health care system are interdependent, enhanced consumer knowledge is perhaps the single most important feature in such a system. The implications of this condi-

---

^{†††}The National Practitioner Data Base is a result of the Health Care Quality Improvement Act, which passed in 1986 and took effect in 1990. From 1990 to 1994, 69,000 health professionals were included in the database. While the National Practitioner Data Base illustrates the restricted access to information that consumers currently have, it is important to note that there are several good, as well as bad, reasons for restricting consumer access. Without appropriate disclaimers and other mitigating circumstances, it is sometimes difficult to interpret what some adverse actions really mean.

tion for an outcome-oriented medical rehabilitation practice, marketing, and financing are enormous. They are discussed later in this chapter.

Conditions Idiosyncratic to Health Care

As noted earlier, one of the key ways in which provider- and payer-driven systems compete today is on the basis of risk: the risk that individuals or groups are likely to be high users of health care services. In a genuine consumer-driven marketplace, risk will be eliminated or minimized as a consideration in the marketing and pricing of health plans. In other words, health markets will be made risk-neutral.

There are several ways in which health markets will be made more risk-neutral. Two of the conditions mentioned as important to facilitating consumer clout in the marketplace are also important to making the market more risk-neutral: (1) making providers price takers through the development of large purchasing groups in which high users are averaged in with low users (Condition 1) and (2) creating a homogeneous product through the development of a standard benefit package that will eliminate the ability of health plans to tweak their benefit packages in an effort to attract lower-risk subscribers (Condition 2).

Two additional conditions are needed to make the health care system more risk-neutral, namely, the use of community ratings (Condition 4) and the use of risk adjusters (Condition 5).

Finally we introduce one last condition, namely consumer governance of the health care system (Condition 6), as a vital element in the creation of a consumer-directed system.

4. Community rating: Health plan premiums are community rated. As noted, one of the ways in which health plans currently compete on risk is by pricing their products on the basis of past and probable future health care utilization. The use of experience ratings discriminates against individuals and groups who are prone to be higher users of health care because of an existing health condition that may require ongoing medical management.

In a consumer-driven health care system, health plans will be available at a community-rated price regardless of the subscriber's health profile or utilization experience. Community rating enables the consumer to have clout in a market that would otherwise be financially inaccessible. Even with community-rated pricing, it will remain necessary, at least in

the early years of such a system, to adjust for the age mix of the subscriber pool.###

The use of community ratings will be essential to the future of medical
rehabilitation, which serves a high-cost user group and whose own labor-
intensive services can be quite expensive. Payer-driven systems that
compete on risk, as well as price, are known to underserve people with
disabilities such as those who need medical rehabilitation services.

*5. Risk adjustment: Health plans, health providers, and health out-
comes are risk-adjusted to reflect the different case mixes of
patients/consumers.* In the current payer-driven environment, health
plans have strong incentives to market and enroll mainly younger and
healthier subscriber groups. In a community-rated market, the incentive
to attract lower-user groups will become stronger since price differentials
based on experience ratings will have been eliminated or significantly
reduced. To dampen or eliminate any residual risk-based competition,
health plans and health providers will be risk-adjusted on the basis of the
sociodemographic and health profile of the subscriber population. In a
true consumer-driven and risk-neutral health care system, mechanisms
will have to be developed to redistribute premium dollars from lower-
risk plans to higher-risk plans.

Risk or case-mix adjustment will also be an important factor in the
assessment of quality and outcomes across different health plans and
providers. Risk-adjusted outcomes will provide consumers a way to
assess accurately the differential outcomes of health plans and providers.

Risk-adjustment mechanisms in the form of case-mix indices at the
provider level have been under development for many years. In acute
care, for example, diagnosis-related groups (DRGs) have been used as a
basis for hospital payment in the Medicare program. Severity-of-illness
measures have been developed and proposed as a supplement to, or a
substitute for, DRGs. In medical rehabilitation, function related groups
(FRGs) have been proposed as a possible method of payment for inpa-

---

###In a community-rated system in which (1) universal coverage remains unimplemented and (2)
health alliances remain voluntary, younger, healthier people and groups will be prone to opt out of
the system unless the community rating is also age-adjusted. This is alleged to be the experience in
the state of New York. Some estimate that as many as 500,000 people dropped their health insurance
after New York state reforms were introduced. Others dispute this finding and argue that the drop off
occurred for other reasons. Modified reforms in Vermont and New Jersey appear to have had the
opposite effect. Bills in the last days of the 103 Congress (i.e., the Mitchell bill and the so-called
mainstream bill [Chafee and Breaux]) do not have pure community rating and provide rate variations
for age of at least 2:1.

tient medical rehabilitation. These case-mix indices, while mainly developed with hospital-based payment in mind, can sometimes also be used to risk-adjust provider outcomes.

Risk-adjustment methodologies at the health-plan level, however, are still in their infancy and will be one of the last features to be implemented fully in a consumer-driven health care system. The lack of a sound risk adjustment at the health plan level may prove to be the Achilles' heel of future health care reform proposals that seek to establish a more level playing field. Until more adequate risk-adjusters are developed, we can expect to see very crude risk adjusters based on sociodemographic factors such as age and gender.

6. Consumer governance: The demand side of the market, that is, consumers and purchasers, dominate the governance of the health care system. In today's health care system, providers and payers are better organized and are dominant players in the political process that shapes American health policy. For evidence of this observation, one has to look no further than the 1993–94 health care reform debate. Indeed, some consumer groups (e.g., the American Association of Retired Persons [AARP]) are organized, but few have the lobbying and media resources that providers and payers can marshal. The 1993–94 health care reform debate was about moving toward a more consumer-directed health care system, a move that will eventually redistribute the roles of providers, payers, and consumers in the governance of the health care system. While the shift toward a more consumer-governed health care system was halted, the long-term shift to greater consumer governance remains a political inevitability.

American health politics, as currently organized, are not a level playing field. In conventional political theory, strong forces in the political process eventually beget strong countervailing forces. This has yet to happen in American health politics. Over time, we will see new consumer-oriented governing boards at the state and federal levels that will supervise the formation of purchasing groups, the definition of benefit packages, the reporting of outcome data, the development of community rating systems, and the implementation of fair risk adjusters. Providers and payers will have an important role in making sure that proposed policies and methodologies are practical and implementable, but their role will be largely advisory to various emerging governing boards in the system.

Managing the Competition

As our health care system attains these six conditions we will begin to see the development of a genuine market-based health care system that competes on price *and quality.* Today's health care markets are most imperfect because they violate *all* the assumptions of "perfect competition." Imperfect markets require rules and supervision to make sure that the participants play fairly on a level playing field. In other words, if there is to be healthy competition in health care, it will have to be managed—more so than other sectors of the American economy. As these six conditions are attained, we will see the implementation of mechanisms to make sure that market participants "play by the rules." The current market is not self-correcting, hence the need for health care reform, which will come either comprehensively or, more likely, incrementally.

A good, but not perfect analogy for market supervision in health care is the role of the Securities and Exchange Commission (SEC), which was established after the 1929 stock market crash to create and govern fair trading practices in the stock and bond markets. The SEC investigates insider trading and has many reporting rules. Stock and bond markets are complicated markets with complicated products not easily understood by the ordinary investor. To simplify matters, for example, the securities market uses risk-adjusters, known as bond ratings (e.g., AAA, BB), that provide a shorthand way for buyers to evaluate probable risk and outcome. Members of the SEC are not allowed to be players in the financial markets they supervise. The SEC is credited for the efficient manner in which American equities and securities markets operate, and for engendering an "… equity market … widely respected as being the broadest, most active, and fairest anywhere." [35] ****

****In the words of Bhide:

> Without doubt, US stock markets are the envy of the world. In contrast to markets in countries such as Germany, Japan, and Switzerland … US equity markets are widely respected as being the broadest, most active, and fairest anywhere. The Securities and Exchange Commission strives mightily to keep them that way. Thanks to the SEC's efforts, trading costs in the US are half those of any other market … The average American, too, can trade with little fear of rigged markets or insider dealings … Wall Street's financiers, who argue passionately for free enterprise, in fact owe a great and unacknowledged debt to their regulators … The historical evidence suggests that, without regulation, stock markets would be marginal institutions.

The regulatory success of the SEC does have its downside, however. The prohibition of insider trading, for example, creates an arm's-length relationship between investors and managers and precludes effective long-term supervision of firms by distant, diffused, outside investors.

IMPLICATIONS FOR OUTCOMES MANAGEMENT IN MEDICAL REHABILITATION

Outcomes will be central to the marketing, pricing, and evaluation of medical rehabilitation services in a consumer-driven health care system. Outcomes are becoming important in the current payer-driven system, but outcome disclosure is selective, is not risk-adjusted, and remains vulnerable to provider gaming. Moreover, rehabilitation outcomes have yet to be used at the health-plan level to enable consumers to make informed health-plan purchasing decisions. The payer-driven interest in outcome management will give way to a more consumer-driven set of outcomes that are publicly disclosed, risk-adjusted, protected from provider gaming, and applicable at the health-plan level as well as the provider level.

Role of Outcome Measurement in Medical Rehabilitation

Medical rehabilitation has had a long-standing interest in functional status and outcome measurement that will serve the field well as the health care system moves toward a genuine competitive market system in which outcomes are central. Outcomes research in medical rehabilitation did not originate with consumer-driven concerns in mind. In earlier days, when medical rehabilitation was largely provider-driven, one important purpose of functional status and outcome measurement was to provide a basis for the field's scientific legitimacy within the larger health sciences community. In the current payer-driven environment, the role of medical rehabilitation outcomes research and management among individual providers is to establish their basic credibility with payers and to justify payment. For traditional inpatient providers, outcomes management helps to demonstrate that, while they have higher costs, they also have superior outcomes.

Scope of Outcome Measurement in Medical Rehabilitation

Medical rehabilitation is fortunate to have already a variety of outcome measures that can be used to evaluate provider performance. The Functional Independence Measure (FIM)[36] and the Patient Evaluation and Conference System (PECS)[37] are two examples of widely accepted measures of functional status and outcome in medical rehabilitation. While they are well accepted, there is a perceived need to look beyond functional status to include issues of social role and community integration. The Craig Handicap Assessment and Reporting Technique (CHART)[38] and Community Integration Survey (CIS)[39] are two examples of such measures.

A key outcome issue in medical rehabilitation is the duration of the postrehabilitation period under review. As one moves beyond the initial rehabilitation episode, the issues of functional status become secondary to the issues of social role and community integration. In a consumer-driven system, these longer-term considerations will become more important. Just how important will be intricately linked to how medical rehabilitation is financed in a consumer-driven system, a topic discussed later.

Risk Adjustment of Medical Rehabilitation Outcomes

Medical rehabilitation is beginning to develop case-mix indices that can be used to risk-adjust outcomes across facilities. A case-mix index such as the FRGs cited earlier was originally intended to help develop a prospective payment system for medical rehabilitation as an analog to the Medicare DRGs used in acute care. Their real importance may be their ability to contribute to a risk-adjustment methodology for evaluating inpatient medical rehabilitation outcomes.[††††] Case-mix and risk-adjustment methodologies that can be applied across rehabilitation settings and modalities have yet to be developed.

Relation to More Generic Measures of Health Outcome

Eventually, in a more consumer-driven system, medical rehabilitation will also have to express its outcomes in more generic terms at the health-plan or provider-network level. One example of a more generic health status survey instrument is the widely mentioned SF-36, a 36-item questionnaire used to assess a person's physical, emotional, functional, and overall health status.[40–42] In other words, medical rehabilitation will have to demonstrate its contribution to the overall well-being or outcomes of a larger consumer group served by a plan or network. Rehabilitation providers will have to be able to explain how their services contribute to the outcomes (risk-adjusted, of course) that are used to

---

††††FIM-based FRGs are calibrated on resource utilization, that is, on length of stay, not on outcomes. Outcomes, in the form of FIM gains, may vary considerably from one impairment group to another.

score entire health plans and shape the ratings used by consumers when making a plan purchasing decision.

Public Disclosure of Medical Rehabilitation Outcome Data

In a consumer-driven, market-based health care system, outcomes and case-mix data at the provider level will become public information. Currently, most providers insist on complete confidentiality regarding their *facility's* performance. In Medical Rehabilitation, for example, data submitted to the National Spinal Cord Injury Data Base (in which model spinal cord injury centers participate) or to the database maintained by the Uniform Data System for Medical Rehabilitation (UDS$_{MR}$) are considered confidential. This policy bars access not only to individual patient records, as it should, but also to any data that can be used to identify providers and evaluate provider performance. Provider confidentiality reflects the high value that our system continues to place on provider autonomy even though the vast majority of medical rehabilitation services are paid for from public funds.

Provider confidentiality, which had its origins in the values of a more provider-driven health care system, is eroding under the pressures of the current payer-driven system and will be eliminated in a consumer-driven system. In the current payer-driven environment, providers are prone to disclose their outcome data when they believe it is to their competitive advantage to do so. Thus, in a payer-driven environment, the disclosure of outcome data tends to be selective, unadjusted for risk (unless the provider is determined to show that its patients have more severe impairments), and difficult to evaluate in the absence of standardized public disclosure requirements. In a consumer-driven system, which is governed in part by the perfect-knowledge assumption of perfect competition, consumers will have access to standardized outcome data that are also risk-adjusted for case mix. Such disclosure and access are essential to a system in which competition is based on price and quality.[‡‡‡‡, §§§§]

[‡‡‡‡] It should be underscored that patient-level data that include personal identifiers or can be traced back to individual patients should remain confidential in a consumer-driven health care system.

[§§§§] If recent experiences are an indicator, health plans and providers will be prone to resist full disclosure of satisfaction and outcomes. The Center for the Study of Services attempted to gather member-satisfaction ratings on 250 health plans used by federal employees, but 60 of the plans would not allow their members to answer the center's questionnaire. In New York, a magazine published risk-adjusted outcome data on coronary artery bypass surgery but was blasted by one hospital administrator as being "anti-doctor and anti-hospital."

In order to achieve data reliability and standardization, all outcome and case-mix data will be subject to audits in order to discourage cheating. In a consumer-driven system where quality, that is, outcome, is a driving force, there will be enormous pressure to rate patients low at admission for purposes of measuring case mix and to rate patients high at discharge and follow-up evaluation for purposes of measuring outcome. Audits at the provider level are likely to be instituted to discourage gaming and to ensure the integrity of a consumer knowledge-based system.

IMPLICATIONS FOR PURCHASING/FINANCING OF MEDICAL REHABILITATION

A consumer-driven, outcomes-based health care system will have profound implications for how we purchase and pay for medical rehabilitation services. In the provider-driven era, which is now passing, inpatient rehabilitation, as noted earlier, has been financed retrospectively by using cost-based methods subject to certain limits under TEFRA for patients with Medicare coverage. TEFRA limits are an example of payer-driven constraints placed on a provider-driven payment system. These limits have proved to be inequitable for hospital providers and are thought to induce unwanted provider behaviors.[23] The proposed use of an FRG-based system, as an alternative to TEFRA, though developed within the field of medical rehabilitation, is essentially an example of a payer-driven approach to medical rehabilitation finance since it is motivated by the payer's, that is, Medicare's, desire to contain costs through a prospective payment system. As noted earlier, managed care, another payer-driven financing approach, is already inducing significant changes in how medical rehabilitation is purchased and delivered in certain markets.

As payer-driven methods of financing, neither FRGs nor managed care (as currently arranged) adequately address the issue of outcomes as an integral part of the rehabilitation purchasing decision and therefore will not survive over the long term, in their current or proposed forms, as the basis of payment in a more consumer-driven, outcomes-based health care system. Payer-driven financing methods should be viewed as part of a longer-term transition to a more outcomes-oriented method of rehabilitation financing.

Selecting Health Plans and Providers

What then might an outcomes-oriented method of purchasing and financing medical rehabilitation services look like in a consumer-driven health care environment? We begin by considering how consumers will choose health plans that include rehabilitation services. One of the great challenges facing medical rehabilitation in a consumer-driven health care system is how to reach out to, and communicate with, the consumer who is making a health plan choice. Most consumers, especially younger ones, never envision a need for medical rehabilitation services, and many will not even know what these services are. The need for medical rehabilitation services is often considered by the average consumer to be a remote possibility and, as such, will not be carefully scrutinized by the consumer when making a health plan decision. Thus, consumers are not likely to make much of an investment in learning about rehabilitation and the quality of various providers within plans when making a health-plan choice.

This state of affairs will require four actions of the medical rehabilitation industry. *First,* the industry will need to develop, in collaboration with a more neutral entity, a single standardized rehabilitation score (with possible subscores) by which health plans will be rated on the basis of the capabilities and performance of the plan's entire network of rehabilitation providers. Such a score would be largely outcome-based and risk-adjusted; it would also create enormous peer pressure to exclude subpar providers and encourage collaboration in helping to improve the plan's overall rehabilitation score. *Second,* the industry will have to convince various health system governing boards and health insurance purchasing cooperatives that a rehabilitation rating system is needed to help consumers make their annual side-by-side comparison of competing health plans. Without such a rating, consumers will overlook the rehabilitation component of a health plan and health plans may not be adequately motivated to include the best possible network of rehabilitation providers. *Third,* the industry will have to adopt the single-score concept (with possible subscores) as the basis for rating individual providers. Such ratings would guide consumers, physician gatekeepers, and health plan case managers in selecting a within-plan or out-of-plan provider when a rehabilitation need arises. And *fourth,* the medical rehabilitation industry will have to undertake an education strategy to inform consumers, physician gatekeepers, and case managers what rehabilitation scores or ratings mean for the choices they need to make when choosing a plan or selecting a provider.[§§, ##]

Financing and Interdisciplinary Medical Rehabilitation

When evaluating the impact of medical rehabilitation, it is often difficult to determine the contribution that each individual component makes to patient outcomes. Rehabilitation practitioners argue that the rehabilitation process is an interdisciplinary one and that the whole is greater than the sum of its parts. The provider-driven method of financing in which rehabilitation services are partitioned into, and billed by, discipline-specific service units undermines the very foundation of interdisciplinary medical rehabilitation so vigorously advocated by rehabilitationists.[####]

Interdisciplinary medical rehabilitation will gain new strength in a consumer-driven outcomes-oriented health care system mainly because of the way in which medical rehabilitation services will be purchased and financed. It is conceivable, for example, that, in the future, health plans and health purchasing cooperatives will purchase medical rehabilitation on a patient-by-patient basis asking different providers within a market area to offer bids in response to a request for proposal (RFP) in which the patient's medical history is profiled and in which certain out-

[§§]A rating system such as the one outlined here will require collaboration among organizations such as the Uniform Data System for Medical Rehabilitation (UDS$_{MR}$) and the Commission on Accreditation of Rehabilitation Facilities (CARF). UDS$_{MR}$, for example, might well become the principal provider of standardized performance data and CARF will likely become the principal evaluator of provider capabilities. We believe that, in a consumer-driven health care system, the role of CARF, for example, will shift from its conventional accreditation function to the additional role of producer of standardized data on which provider capabilities will be evaluated and translated for consumer consumption.

[##]The consumer-driven medical rehabilitation assessment system envisioned here will also come to replace the physician-based assessment used by organizations such as the US News and World Report in conducting its annual survey of the ten best rehabilitation hospitals. Such surveys are based largely on physician-peer perceptions that are shaped less by the provider's quality of patient care and more by the provider's academic and research prowess and by the provider's marketing and public relations capabilities.

[####]In fact it could be argued that medical rehabilitation, by disaggregating services into billable, discipline-specific units, is pricing the concept of interdisciplinary medical rehabilitation out of existence and is bringing the demise of interdisciplinary rehabilitation upon itself.

comes are specified.***** The lowest bidder will provide any combination or bundle of services (e.g., physical therapy, speech and language, home health, durable medical equipment) the provider considers necessary to achieve a particular set of outcomes most efficiently.†††††, ‡‡‡‡‡ This bundling will encourage interdisciplinary collaboration. There will be no attempt to disaggregate all the different services, and providers will be free to reallocate services and resources as needed to achieve the predetermined set of outcomes.§§§§§ In order to encourage provider participation, the offeror might agree to share some of the financial risk with the provider, especially in those cases where the probable long-term outcome is too difficult to predict. Payment will be contingent on completion of predetermined outcomes at the end of a designated period such as 6 months. Staged payments to reflect work in progress and various post-rehabilitation outcomes may also be devised.

This kind of financing will help to terminate the endless disputes about whether the service in question was covered, whether the service was justified, or whether the patient was hospitalized too long. Payers, including managed care plans, will no longer serve as "health police" and micromanage providers. In short, such a system will restore some of the provider autonomy that is being lost in payer-driven health care. Such a system may also induce the creation of a brokerage function in which firms specializing in RFP development and case management will provide highly specialized brokerage services or may themselves assume risk for outcome and costs.¶¶¶¶¶

*****In a system that is fully consumer-driven, the outcomes listed in the RFP would be identified jointly with the patient or a family member. Such a plan could encourage greater patient ownership of the rehabilitation process and encourage more vigorous participation. In some instances, probable outcomes are not always known. Moreover, upon onset of a major disabling impairment, patients or families may not always be in a position to grasp the options that lie ahead fully.

†††††If the consumer or family prefers a more expensive provider, they would pay out-of-pocket for the difference.

‡‡‡‡‡The bundling of rehabilitation services envisioned here should not be confused with the bundling concepts proposed by others such as Kane and Neu who have proposed to bundle a greater range of postacute care services, the need for which would be determined by acute care providers.

§§§§§Our vision for the future of an outcomes-oriented method of financing medical rehabilitation services was stimulated by Robert Magnuson, who has proposed an RFP bidding process for medical rehabilitation services.

¶¶¶¶¶One example of an at-risk broker is California-based Paradigm, Inc., which provides brokerage services between payers and providers for people with brain injuries who need rehabilitation services. Largely a workers' compensation product, the Paradigm model could be generalized to other payers who also have long-term financial liability for the rehabilitation and postrehabilitation needs of their subscribers. Paradigm's ability to go at risk for certain predefined outcomes is, in part, the result of an outcomes database that can be used to determine probable outcomes for new cases.

In this kind of financing scenario, the performance of individual providers and brokers will be used to rate overall health plans and individual providers as noted earlier.¶¶¶¶¶

The consumer-driven health care system envisioned here will develop in stages. At the outset, health plans and health purchasing cooperatives will have difficulty knowing how to risk-adjust and price out medical rehabilitation services. Medical rehabilitation patients, such as those seen in inpatient facilities, will be viewed as outliers or high-cost catastrophic cases. In the absence of adequate risk adjusters and cost information, we envision a transition period in which a "carve-out" will be made to treat rehabilitation services and rehabilitation patients separately. Such a carve-out may become a separate program within the Medicare program (e.g., a Part D program) or it may entail a separate allocation of resources within each health insurance purchasing cooperative designed to handle high-cost catastrophic cases akin to a reinsurance mechanism that we find in current plans. A carve-out can accelerate the development of a case-by-case competitive bidding process and provide the utilization-and-cost database that individual health plans and others will use in pricing and marketing the rehabilitation portion of their benefit packages.

CONCLUSION

The road to a consumer-driven health care system is a long one with many potential detours that will depend on how the federal government and the states approach the issue of health care reform in the months and years to come. The road may be a bumpy one especially as health care passes over the bridge of payer-driven health care that is still under construction in many markets across the land. Nonetheless, like distant city lights in the night, many elements of a consumer-driven system can already be seen flickering on the horizon and will shape the route we choose in reaching our destination.

The elements of a consumer-driven system that are already faintly visible include the concept of large health insurance purchasing groups, the

---

¶¶¶¶¶Some of the medical rehabilitation purchasing arrangements envisioned here may not be appropriate for the patient who needs intermittent or lower-level rehabilitation intervention. The process of securing competitive bids is not necessarily efficient below certain thresholds of anticipated costs. For such individuals, usually treated on an outpatient basis, purchasing decisions will probably be made by consumers and their gatekeeping physicians using provider ratings and consumer satisfaction scores of those rehabilitation providers included in the health plan.

notion of a standard benefit package, the need for community rating, and the development of risk adjusters and case-mix indices. The elements already very visible are the move to make providers price takers, the use of consumer satisfaction surveys, and, above all, the health outcomes movement that is so central to the consumer knowledge assumption of competitive markets theory.

Medical rehabilitation has many well-placed provisions for the journey ahead, especially its long-standing commitment to outcomes research. The field has been largely unprepared for the stormy weather of the managed care revolution now passing across the country from west to east as most weather patterns do. By looking ahead to the coming consumer revolution in health care, medical rehabilitation should be better prepared for the emerging new order in American health care.

REFERENCES

1. Meili P. The rehabilitation market. *Rehabil Manage*. April/May 1993:96–102.

2. Wolk S, Blair T. *Trends in Medical Rehabilitation*. Reston, Va: American Rehabilitation Association; 1994.

3. Melvin J, Zollar C, eds. *Access Rehabilitation: A Focus for the Health Care Reform Debate*. Washington, DC: National Association of Rehabilitation Facilities; 1993.

4. National Institutes of Health. *Research Plan for the National Center for Medical Rehabilitation Research*. U.S. Department of Health Services; 1993.

5. Granger C, Hamilton B. The Uniform Data System for Medical Rehabilitation Report of First Admissions for 1992. *Am J Phys Med Rehabil*. 1994;73(1):51–55.

6. Kottke F, Knapp M. The development of physiatry before 1950. *Arch Phys Med Rehabil*. 1988;69:4–14.

7. Pope A, Tarlov A. *Disability in America, toward a National Agenda for Prevention*. Washington, DC: Institute of Medicine, National Academy Press; 1991.

8. Rice D, La Plante M. Medical expenditures for disability and disabling conditions. *Am J Public Health*. 1992;82 (5):739–741.

9. National Center for Health Statistics. *Health, United States, 1993*. Hyattsville, Md: Public Health Service; 1994.

10. Gruenberg E. The failures of success. *Milbank Q*. 1977;55(1):3–24.

11. DeJong G. Number of adults with severe disabilities has grown. *Bus Health*. 1987;4.

12. Verbrugge L. Longer life but worsening health? Trends in health and mortality of middle aged and older persons. *Milbank Q*. 1984;62(3):450–484.

13. Prospective Payment Assessment Commission. (1992). *Medicare and the American Health Care System, Report to Congress*.

14. Batavia A. *The Payment of Medical Rehabilitation Services: Current Mechanisms and Potential Models*. Chicago: American Hospital Association; 1988.

15. Neu C, Harrison S, Heilburn J. *Medicare Patients and Postacute Care*. Santa Monica, Calif: RAND.

16. Ross B. The impact of reimbursement issues on rehabilitation nursing practice and patient care. *Rehabil Nurs.* 1992;17(5):236–238.

17. Saunders W. Overview. *Health Care Financ Rev.* 1993;15 (2):1–5.

18. Arqueta A, Lakin C, Hill B. (1991). Persons in institutions and special settings. In: Thompson Hoffmans, Storck I, eds. *Disability in the United States: A Portrait from National Data.* New York: Springer Publishing; 1991:184–208.

19. Marion Merrell Dow. *Managed Care Digest, HMO Edition.* Kansas City: Marion Merrell Dow Inc; 1994.

20. Kertesz L. A blue streak for managed care. *Mod Health Care.*1994;24(37):63–66, 68,70.

21. Foster Higgins. *National Survey of Employer Sponsored Health Plans.* New York.

22. Batavia A, DeJong G. Prospective payment for medical rehabilitation: The DHHS report to Congress. *Arch Phys Med Rehabil.* 1988;69(5):377–380.

23. Langenbrunner J, Willis P, Jencks S, et al. Developing payment refinements and reforms under Medicare for excluded hospitals. *Health Care Financ Rev* 1989;10:91–107.

24. Wilkerson D, Batavia A, DeJong G. Use of functional status measures for payment of medical rehabilitation services. *Arch Phys Med Rehabil.* 1992;73 (2):111–120.

25. Harada N, Sofaer S, Kominski G. Functional status outcomes in rehabilitation: implications for prospective payment. *Med Care.* 1993;31(4):345–357.

26. Stineman M, Escarce J, Goin J, et al. A case-mix classification system for medical rehabilitation. *Med Care.* 1994;32(4):366–379.

27. Tepper S, DeJong G, Wilkerson D, Brannon R. (1995). Criteria for the selection of a payment methodology for inpatient medical rehabilitation. *Arch of Phys Med Rehabil.* Forthcoming.

28. Prospective Payment Assessment Commission. *Report and Recommendations to the Congress, March 1, 1994.*

29. American Hospital Association. *Survey of Medical Rehabilitation Hospitals and Programs—1991.* Chicago: American Hospital Association; 1993.

30. McMillan A. Trends in Medicare health maintenance organization enrollment: 1986–93. *Health Care Financ Rev.* 1993;15(1):135–146.

31. Marion Merrell Dow. *Managed Care Digest, Long Term Care Edition.* Kansas City: Marion Merrell Dow Inc; 1994.

32. Coile R. (1994). Forecasting the future. *Rehabil Manage.* December/January 1994:53–55.

33. de LaFuente D. For-profit chains' growth helps boost rehab industry. *Mod Health Care.* 1993;23(21):58–62.

34. Preister R. A values framework for health system reform. *Health Affairs.* 1992;11(1):84–107.

35. Bhide A. Efficient markets, deficient governance. *Harvard Bus Rev.* 1994;72(6):129–139.

36. Hamilton B, Granger C, Sherwin F, Zielezny M, Tashman J. A uniform national data system for medical rehabilitation. In: Fuhrer M, ed. *Rehabilitation Outcomes: Analysis and Measurement.* Baltimore: Paul H. Brookes Publishing Co; 1987.

37. Harvey R, Jellinek H. Patient profiles: utilization in functional performance assessment. *Arch Phys Med Rehabil.* 1983;64:268–271.

38. Whiteneck G, Charlifue S, Gerhart K, Overholser J, Richardson G. Quantifying handicap: a measure of long-term rehabilitation outcomes. *Arch Phys Med Rehabil.* 1992;73(6):519–526.

39. Willer B, Rosenthal M, Kreutzer J, Gordon W, Rimpel R. Assessment of community integration following rehabilitation for traumatic brain injury. *J Head Trauma Rehabil.* 1993;8(2):75–87.

40. Ware J, Sherbourne C. The MOS 36-item Short Form Health Survey (SF-36), conceptual framework and item selection. *Med Care.* 1992;30(6):473–483.

41. Hays R, Shapiro M. (1992). An overview of generic health related quality of life measures for HIV research. *Quality Life Res.* 1992;1:91–97.

42. Stewart A, Ware J. *Measuring Functioning and Well-Being: The Medical Outcomes Study Approach.* Durham, NC: Duke University Press; 1992.

Chapter 2

Conceptualizing
Clinical Outcomes

D. Nathan Cope, MD, and Paula Sundance, MD

Objectives

- To define case conceptualization and clinical outcome.
- To present a model that distinguishes among five outcome levels that range along a continuum from medical instability to productive activity.
- To demonstrate how clinical outcome levels can be used effectively in patient management.

In our current state of national scrutiny of health policy and cost-effectiveness, the value of an outcomes approach to rehabilitation is obvious. Outcome-oriented rehabilitation fundamentally includes the identification of appropriate clinical outcomes for persons served and the measurement of these outcomes to determine if they have been achieved. Equally important to this process is determining how these outcomes can be achieved in a resource-wise, or cost-effective manner. There is widespread if not universal acceptance of the need for improved resource allocation for health care services based upon empirical data-driven outcome analyses. It has become unacceptable to base treatment decisions in rehabilitation, as well as in more acute medical phases of care, upon "clinical opinion" or other basically anecdotal processes. In this chapter we will present a conceptual model of outcome management and an operational structure that can be used to organize clinical outcomes consistently along a continuum of care. We will suggest how these outcomes can be measured validly and reliably. Finally, we will address how this approach can contribute to a more cost-effective health care system.

For purposes of clarity, it is important at this point to establish some specific definitions of the term *outcome*. These are presented in Table 2–1.

Table 2–1 Definitions of Outcomes

Global Outcome	The global outcome is the end result of all clinical issues and treatments expressed in the most general form. It is the result of "patient-specific outcomes," residual impairments, disabilities, and handicaps. It is an expression of the objective recovery achieved and the subjective perceptions experienced that contribute to a person's quality of life.
Outcome Levels	Outcome levels are specific categories or groupings of patient problems and conditions that typically occur in the course of rehabilitation and recovery. Examples include achievement of physiologic stability, establishment in the residential environment, and return to productive activity. There are six outcome levels, ranging from 0 to V (presented in this chapter.)
Patient-Specific Outcomes	Patient-specific outcomes are the individual goals achieved through recovery and treatment of identified problems specific to the patient and clinical condition. These may be medical, functional, psychological, social, or vocational in nature. The collective result of achieving a group of patient-specific outcomes is typically the achievement of an outcome level.

A rehabilitation process driven by appropriate outcomes has a variety of benefits. This system allows patients in any phase of treatment, from acute injury or illness through complete reintegration into society and work, to be operationally described and classified. It allows for the allocation of resources and the cost accounting of resources to various "phases" of care. This system links specific treatment paths to resource utilization. It thus serves as a foundation upon which specific treatment interventions regarding appropriateness and cost-effectiveness can be arranged and evaluated.

When a clinician or treatment team approaches the clinical situation of a catastrophically injured or ill patient, with intentions of developing a logical and comprehensive rehabilitation treatment plan, the large number of distinct issues that require attention and resolution in order to achieve a "successful" result or outcome becomes evident. Management of patients recovering from catastrophic loss is complex. The traditional problem-oriented approach has value in defining and approaching problems but has limitations relative to the establishment of a continuum of care. Another risk of this traditional approach is that important issues go unaddressed or are addressed in a less than optimal order. The result can be incomplete and poor global outcomes or excessive time and resource consumption to achieve target outcomes. Outcome-oriented case conceptualization allows for a more complete perspective relative to the appropriate global outcome. With conceptualization of outcome, the sequence of problem resolution or treatment to achieve this global result most efficiently, can be reverse-engineered. The clinical ability to conceptualize the entirety of a case at the beginning of care traditionally comes from experience with a large number of cases as well as the opportunity to follow these cases over an extended period of years. This extended period of observation brings a valid appreciation of the relevant factors producing durability of result that cannot be fully appreciated with only a limited view of each patient. Although such conceptual ability cannot really be achieved by a clinician without time and experience, it is necessary to bring the proper conceptual perspective to these cases if one is to avoid a career of making short-term treatment interventions over many cases and over many years without feedback regarding long-term impact. Thus it is important to learn to view each case from the "end point backward," that is, first to visualize the optimal reasonable achievable global outcome goal and then to reverse-engineer the sequence of treatments necessary to arrive at that global result.

An outcome-driven system should be able to operationally define what constitutes an optimal global outcome. To state a global outcome in qualitative terms such as returning a patient to "as able-bodied a functional state as possible" or "maximum independence" is really to state not much at all. It is nearly impossible to make logical analyses of the contribution any individual treatment intervention would make to such a nonspecifically described outcome. Multiple treatments, each more or less relevant, could be equally encompassed under such a nonspecific structure. True, it is common in rehabilitation to operationalize many treatment goals, such as "The patient will be able to ambulate over all terrain with stand-by assistance." Nevertheless, in the authors' experience when one moves from these "microgoals" to more global outcome statements, a more qualitative type of statement becomes the rule. For example, a program to reduce a contracture through prolonged stretch, ultrasound, and so on, could conceivably contribute equally well to achieving "as able-bodied a functional state as possible" regardless of whether the contracture contributed in a meaningful way to achieving a significant global outcome. Outcomes described in a nonspecific manner have limited ability to structure a treatment logic upon the course of care. It is essential to impose a treatment logic and hierarchy of process upon the many potential clinical problems and treatments relating to each case. Only after such global outcomes can be visualized and articulated (ideally in written discrete operational terms) does it become possible to establish a system of communication and responsibility in which all participants (clinicians, patient, family, payers, etc.) can understand their contribution and accountability. Operationalizing the ultimate global results being sought is the important first step in an outcome-oriented rehabilitation process. The process of creating such operationalized definitions will be further discussed later.

It seems obvious, but bears emphasis at this point, *that not all problems and not all treatment goals are equal.* It is a primary task of the clinician to sort and prioritize these problems. Some problems are critical in both the rapidity with which they must be addressed and the relative impact with which their solution will have on an overall outcome. Other problems may be better and more effectively addressed at a later stage of treatment. Some problems and goals may, when viewed through a reverse-engineering model, not require significant attention at all if they are not going to impact the overall global result sought.

OUTCOME LEVELS

Outcome levels represent the basic domains that human beings include in their lives, such as health, personal maintenance, home management, community activities, and productivity. With catastrophic illness or injury, an individual typically becomes disabled to varying degrees relative to each of these domains. With the process of healing and adaptation to the residual impairments and disabilities, the person who has experienced catastrophic loss recovers varying levels of functional independence within each of these domains. It is useful to analyze the entire spectrum of any patient's clinical issues by establishing in which outcome level the specific problems and treatments appropriately reside. The individual's associated outcome level in the clinical and rehabilitation recovery continuum is identified by this process, which also defines the most immediately appropriate specific treatments to implement. Outcome levels typically involve a related site of care (e.g., for physiologic instability a hospital is a usual site). Nevertheless, outcome level is not defined by the site of care, but rather by the nature of the typical clinical issues being addressed.

Determining within which outcome level an individual patient lies establishes the general types and outcomes appropriate for that patient at that point in the continuum of treatment. This determination gives focus and temporal organization to the typically large and complex list of possible treatments for that patient. A schema of clinical outcome levels is presented in Exhibit 2–1. The authors have successfully used this model to conceptualize the continuum of treatment interventions and of nodal points in the process. There are six clinical outcome levels.

Exhibit 2–1 Outcome Levels 0–V

0 = physiologic instability
I = physiologic stability
II = physiologic maintenance
III = residential reintegration
IV = community reintegration
V = productive activity
Source: Copyright ©1993, Paradigm Health Corporation.

Level 0: Physiologic Instability

Physiologic instability means that medical and physiologic conditions have not yet been completely assessed, diagnosed, and managed, irrespective of a patient's site of treatment. Although not an outcome level per se, the category of physiologic instability is most often used to describe patients as they first appear after onset of their injury or illness. These patients are most frequently, but not universally, cared for within the acute hospital care system. Patients at this level have unmanaged acute medical diagnostic and management problems that usually mandate that they receive care in an acute care setting, that is, a hospital, or an intensive care unit (ICU), or an acute medical/surgical ward. A patient who has just experienced a major trauma and is in an ICU, who is hemodynamically unstable, for example, is at this level. It is possible, however, that a patient at this level may be at a different site of care. The patient who has grade III pressure sore and is living at home may also be physiologically unstable until medical diagnostic evaluations are complete and a treatment program that allows the pressure sore to heal has begun. A patient with a neurogenic bladder that it is being suboptimally managed as evidenced by frequent urinary tract infections is physiologically unstable until appropriate assessments, interventions, and management strategies have been established.

Level I: Physiologic Stability

Physiologic stability is the first and most basic clinical outcome level. It is achieved when all major medical and physiologic problems have been addressed and are being appropriately managed. No major volatile or undiagnosed symptoms remain. Typically all major medical issues have been resolved to the extent that discharge from an acute hospital setting is clinically appropriate. With the achievement of physiologic stability, the altered clinical systems residual to catastrophic loss have appropriate management strategies established, including clinically indicated treatment, monitoring, and maintenance protocols. There may be active medical and surgical conditions remaining, but management strategies have been established that allow for discharge from the acute hospital facility and do not require intensive physician and/or nursing management.

Example

For a case of severe burn injury, achievement of physiologic stability would imply acute débridement and skin coverage procedures have been completed; hemodynamic, respiratory, and metabolic complications resolved; and diagnosis and management of sequelae established. However, the patient may still require splinting and protective garments and may face future reconstructive surgical procedures.

Example

For a case of multiple long bone trauma, achievement of physiologic stability would imply that all acute fractures have been definitively diagnosed, stabilized, and healing without evidence of other physiologic system complications. The patient may use a cast with weight-bearing restrictions.

Appropriate rehabilitation services at the physiologic stability clinical outcome are coincidental to, but may occur in parallel with, the basic acute medical and surgical care of the patient. These rehabilitation services may include establishment of long-term management strategies for altered clinical systems, preventative therapy (e.g., skin and joint preservation activities), evaluations, identification of and referral to appropriate rehabilitation or other treatment management resources, and planning of future care needs. Although a varying amount of functional restoration may be achieved in parallel with the process of achieving medical stabilizing, such achievements are not considered a part of the physiologic stability clinical outcome level.

Level II: Physiologic Maintenance

The physiologic maintenance clinical outcome level addresses the achievement of basic rehabilitation outcomes that are intrinsically necessary to *preserve* the immediate and long-term physiologic health of the patient. Typically these programs establish adequate and safe systems of nutrition, prevention of aspiration, skin preservation, joint maintenance, bowel and bladder management programs. Functional goals are limited to fundamental domains such as a basic degree of bed mobility, continence, or transfers within the patient's capacity. Only a limited degree of mobility, self-care, communication, and cognitive and behavioral outcomes is necessarily part of this clinical outcome level and only to the extent that such functional achievement directly contributes to physiologic maintenance. Clinical outcomes of physiologic maintenance are typically those achieved within hospital-based acute rehabilitation centers, although aspects of this outcome level may be provided in other settings, including subacute rehabilitation, postacute residential, outpatient, or home settings. This level of outcome does assume the achievement of the necessary functional and management goals in order to discharge the patient safely to a long-term residential (home or other) or postacute residential rehabilitation setting. The specific goals for the individual patient, relative to the physiologic maintenance outcome level, are determined in relation to that patient's capacity.

Example

A patient with a C-5 complete spinal cord injury with unimpaired cognitive function may still be dependent in all mobility and self-care skills after achievement of this outcome level. Achievement of physiologic maintenance clinical outcome might imply, however, that the patient *is* able to direct the care provided by others (family or attendants) relative to physiologic maintenance.

Example

A patient with a T-10 complete spinal cord injury might be expected to achieve an assisted level of independence in self-care and mobility skills at the physiologic maintenance outcome level because of the patient's greater capacity for this level of independence.

Level III: Primary Functional Goals— Home and/or Residential Integration

Clinical outcome level III refers to moving a patient through all necessary treatment and rehabilitation to achieve a contextually acceptable level of function within the site of a long-term residence (typically the patient's home, although any site of long-term residence, e.g., a nursing home or board-and-care facility, may be involved). Specific goals relative to this clinical outcome include achievement of proficiency in self-care, mobility, communication, safety, and home management to function in that residential setting. The focus of treatment at this clinical outcome level is to allow the patient to function reasonably and safely in the home or other residential setting appropriate for that patient's clinical capacity and residential environmental conditions. Typical goals relative to this clinical outcome would be functional and safe mobility within the home or residential setting, establishment of an effective general communication system, and attainment of functional capability in a variety of personal and home management areas such as self-care, mobility, safety, cooking, light housekeeping, and household planning. It is at this point that the patient and/or family typically may become part of the care and management process by incorporating and taking over those skills and activities required to maintain physiologic stability in the residential setting. This clinical outcome level reflects the clinically appropriate transition and transfer of the patient to the least restrictive long-term environment.

Level IV: Advanced Functional Goals— Community Reintegration

Clinical outcome level IV focuses on achievement of the advanced rehabilitation outcomes necessary to achieve an appropriate level of function within the patient's community. Goals include self-management and social competencies, community mobility, complex homemaking capabilities, financial management, self-directed health monitoring, recreation, and other community activities. This clinical outcome level is usually achieved by treatment delivered within the home and community settings, although some postacute residential and day treatment program involvement may be included. The patient's ultimate handicap relative to community reintegration is dependent upon both the patient's disability and the particular community or environment in which the patient will be required to function. The patient's impairment relative to this clinical outcome level determines the appropriate level of independence or assistance to be targeted. This implies that the availability of assistance and other resources to the patient within his or her community to support such level of community reintegration is a factor included in assessing appropriate goals.

Example
A person with polio who uses a crutch may be more handicapped living in Chicago than San Diego because of inclement weather and more architectural barriers. In this case, the individual's handicap is specific to the community.

Example
For a hemiplegic patient without adequate family support, who will be residing in a nursing home, community reintegration may be limited to establishing connection with whatever supported activities are available in the nursing home. If the patient has appropriate family resources, a much more aggressive community mobility and reintegration program may be appropriate.

Level V: Productive Activity

Clinical outcome level V refers to establishing the individual in productive activities within his or her capacity. These goals should be appropriate to the patient's interests and stage of life: that is, they may involve vocational, avocational, or educational pursuits. For example, productive activity does not necessarily mean return to work. For the pediatric population, productive activity may involve educational reintegration. A typical component of this outcome level is vocational evaluation, including assessments of the individual's education, work history, transferable skills, abilities, impairments, disabilities, interests, and motivation to implement recommendations for a vocational plan. Effective reintegration into productive activity may include a job site analysis and employer education in addition to vocational education, job training, and job coaching. The patient's disability and the employer's capacity determine the level of employment achieved: competitive, modified, sheltered, volunteer. The individual's handicap relative to occupation is dependent upon his or her disability, the job requirements, and the employer's environment.

Example
For a 63-year-old woman who has had a gratifying recovery from a brain injury and has returned to her community there may be no interest in returning to her premorbid employment, but rather a choice of appropriate volunteer activities.

Example
For a 16-year-old burn patient, an appropriate goal may be to return to school with an appropriate individual educational plan.

ORGANIZING PATIENT-SPECIFIC OUTCOMES ALONG A CONTINUUM

In summary, outcome levels are general statements specifying nodal points of the overall clinical and adaptive recovery targeted or achieved relative to the individual patient's capacity. The specific treatments delivered to achieve such general results can be organized around the sequential achievement of each progressive outcome level. Determination of the appropriate clinical outcome level to be addressed at any given stage in recovery organizes the rehabilitation treatment strategies and selection of the most appropriate patient-specific treatments and outcomes. Thus, outcome levels represent points in the continuum of recovery and care from catastrophic loss where patterns or clusters of essential care or management issues should logically be collectively addressed. Clinical outcome levels are hierarchical, proceeding from the most basic level, where medical instability is the essential care issue, through physiologic stabilization, physiologic maintenance, transition to the residential setting, establishment within the community, and return to productive activity. Each clinical outcome level generally presupposes the achievement of all lower level goals.

Example

A burn patient who is medically unstable must achieve *outcome level I: physiologic stability* before he or she has the capacity to pursue the clinical *outcome level II: physiologic maintenance* and return to and be integrated into *outcome level III: the home environment* (or other equivalent).

Example

A person who has had a spinal cord injury, who is physiologically stable, established in the home environment, and appropriately reintegrated into his or her community may be ready for *outcome level V: return to work.*

The authors would assert that it is inefficient to focus upon level III residential or level IV community reintegration before level I or II is achieved. It is similarly inappropriate to expend excessive resources in the acute phase of management addressing issues (specific outcomes) that will not significantly contribute to outcome level achievement within our current health care system. The consequence of doing so may be to have insufficient resources to adequately address level III, IV, or V outcomes.

For each clinical outcome level, a core group of specific issues are typically addressed. Thus patient-specific goals appropriate for level III, appearing in an operational treatment plan focusing on achievement of level II, can be readily identified and given close scrutiny, that is, their appropriateness at that point in the continuum of care can be assessed. Such specific treatments and outcomes that appear out of this logical outcome level sequence can be readily identified and deleted, rescheduled, or otherwise appropriately modified.

Example

For a severely neurologically impaired patient during achievement of outcome level I or II, it is likely to be clinically inappropriate and inefficient to consider work on a complex augmented communication system. It is more clinically appropriate to address such a goal after the medical and basic physiologic conditions have been resolved, when the patient enters the stage of care addressing outcome level III or IV. The patient at this point is more able physically to cooperate, the suitability of the communication system proposed can be judged within the environment in which it must be utilized, and, finally, the relative cost of providing such treatment is usually less in the (typically nonhospital) level III setting than in level I or II care.

In addition, an empirical listing of typical or essential patient-specific outcomes can be derived from experience in achieving any specific level of outcome. Any excessive treatment goals, or any missing critical outcomes, can be identified by reference to the empirical "checklist" of specific outcomes.

Example

To achieve a level II outcome, a patient who has an acute cervical spinal cord injury will need to achieve specific outcomes relating to medical stabilization; nursing protocols in place for skin, bowel, bladder, respiratory care, and so on. He or she will require a variety of educational and counseling outcomes and provision of equipment. It is possible to review this list quickly for completeness and identify further needed components, such as a home evaluation and modification plan to allow discharge to the next planned level of residence and care.

Recovery from catastrophic loss is complex. It can be overwhelming to attempt to prioritize and manage the rehabilitation process comprehensively for individuals who have catastrophic injury or illness with its almost limitless issues and problems. Conceptualizing a catastrophic case relative to a sequential hierarchy of outcome levels simplifies such management strategies. Restricting specific goal setting to include only those relevant to the immediately germane clinical outcome level effectively organizes and prioritizes problems and treatment strategies. (This relegation of tasks to specific outcome levels is not an absolute rule. Many exceptions can be conceived where various factors mandate treatment "out of order." However, the general appreciation of this association of specific outcomes with each outcome level does provide a method for giving explicit scrutiny for treatments and goals that *typically* would not be included in a particular phase of care.)

APPLYING AN OUTCOME LEVEL PARADIGM IN THE DELIVERY OF RESULTS-ORIENTED REHABILITATION

Clinical outcome levels are a valuable way of organizing patient management. They represent nodal points in the process of care and rehabilitation where typical issues of particular types of care or recovery tend to be typically resolved. Clinical outcomes levels are intended to be general statements of the overall medical and rehabilitation recovery achieved by a given patient. Any individual patient, however, will fall only approximately into a clinical outcome level category because of varying rates of recovery and resolution for each specific clinical problem and patient.

Patients may exceed one aspect of a particular area in one outcome level and yet have other aspects that may not be totally resolved.

Each outcome level encompasses a range of the results of medical, functional, psychologic, and social and vocational treatments. There is latitude for structuring varying types of interventions within each outcome level, including traditional medical interventions, such as seizure management with anticonvulsant medication or establishment of a bowel management protocol, and significant social tasks and outcomes, such as establishing a guardianship, providing psychological counseling to a spouse, or establishing advocacy for the patient with community agencies. These types of interventions, although critical to the ultimate success and durability of the overall outcome level, are difficult to get funded because of traditional benefit designs that authorize only certain types of professional services, for example, physician management or nursing care, but perhaps not psychologic assessment and treatment. When a transformation is made so that the benefit design is defined as achievement of a durable outcome level, a significant increase in flexibility of treatment design results.

For example, the role the family is able to play in the support system significantly impacts the outcome and outcome durability of catastrophic loss. Typically, people tend to have the best clinical outcome levels if they have a stable family situation, although there are certainly exceptions to this statement. The authors' clinical experience indicates that the family and other support system of each patient need to be educated, counseled, and empowered as early in the clinical course after catastrophic loss as possible. It is important to include such nonmedical treatments as family education and counseling within the specific outcomes and criteria for achievement of even outcome level I or II, despite the focus of these levels upon physiologic restoration. Yet traditional benefit design currently mandates that these services often are unfunded and thus tend to be underaddressed by providers. To that extent they become an integral component of an outcome level I or II they are funded indistinguishably from all other critical elements of care.

A final benefit of organizing rehabilitation care through the perspective of outcome levels is the capability for finer financial and cost analysis of results. One can look at aggregate samples of particular patient types, matched on salient clinical and other characteristics, and determine typical resource consumption patterns to achieve any specific change in outcome level. For example, one can analyze the average cost of moving a patient with a particular type of disability from an outcome level I to an outcome level II or III. Other statistical descriptors, such as the range, standard deviation, or variance, are also feasible and of interest. This then allows the development of various prospective pricing arrangements for catastrophic rehabilitation, a capability the authors' organization[1] has been utilizing for several years. It also allows analysis of differing providers and varying treatment plans, both to distinguish efficient from inefficient providers and to discover optimal "critical pathways" of care.

REFERENCE

1. Paradigm Health Corp., 1001 Galaxy Way, Suite Number 400, Concord, CA 94520. Telephone: 510/676-2300.

Chapter 3

Outcome Level I: Physiologic Stability—Acute Management

Paula Sundance, MD, and D. Nathan Cope, MD

Objectives

- To define and give clinical examples of the first outcome level, physiological stability.
- To identify the specific, targeted outcomes that are critical to the achievement of outcome level I.
- To demonstrate how the achievement of the first outcome level influences subsequent outcome levels.

In this chapter we focus on the earliest and most fundamental aspect of recovery and rehabilitation—outcome level I, medical or physiologic stability (also see Chapter 2). The intent of this chapter is not to recapitulate principles of acute medical and trauma care; more than adequate texts exist for this purpose. Rather the purpose is to provide a perspective on how an awareness of case conceptualization and an ultimate global outcome with an organized visualization of the total rehabilitation process, even in this very early stage of treatment (when typically attention is principally focused upon resuscitation efforts and patient survival), can significantly contribute to both ultimate outcome and optimization of health care resources. Associated with achieving clinical outcome level I is impelling an efficient and cost-effective coordination of treatments across all subsequent outcome levels (II–V) to achieve an appropriate global clinical result. The intent is to guide the reader's thinking in how to design and implement effective rehabilitation treatments to achieve specific outcome levels along this continuum of care.

OUTCOME LEVEL 0: PHYSIOLOGIC INSTABILITY

The term *physiologic instability* may be used to describe patients' condition as they typically present within the acute medical care system. Patients at this level characteristically have multiple acute medical diagnostic and management conditions that are incompletely defined and managed and usually mandate that they receive care in the acute hospital setting, including within the intensive care unit (ICU) or acute medical or surgical ward. Clearly a patient who has just experienced major trauma and presents to the emergency room with hemodynamic instability is in this category. Evaluation and management of acute life-threatening systems failure proceed intensively and simultaneously. Emergency medical and trauma management systems diagnose and manage life-threatening conditions including circulatory shock, acute respiratory failure, and impaired cellular metabolism.

Example
A patient with major trauma that includes severe brain injury is assessed and managed for life-threatening conditions urgently and simultaneously: (1) The airway and adequate ventilation are established; (2) the assessment for other life-threatening conditions that could lead to death during neurologic evaluation and treatment is initiated; (3) while appropriate precautions are taken, an evaluation for possible concurrent cervical spine injury is completed. With the initiation of life-preserving trauma assessments and management, neurological and imaging evaluations of brain injury proceed. Neurosurgical interventions may limit secondary injury by control of hemorrhage, decompression of brain tissue, and débridement of necrotic tissue and foreign material. An intracranial pressure (ICP) monitor may be placed, allowing for the monitoring of cerebral perfusion pressure, thus facilitating timely and appropriate interventions for decreasing intracerebral pressure to reduce secondary brain injury. In the intensive care unit continuous monitoring and assessments allow for timely and appropriate management strategies designed to support critical systems, preserve function, and minimize secondary injury and complications.

In addition, physiologic instability may also arise or be present in patients in other settings.

Example

An individual in whom a Grade 3 pressure sore has developed while he or she has been living in an extended care facility is physiologically unstable until appropriate medical diagnostic evaluations have been completed and the indicated treatment program that will in the normal course of events allow the pressure sore to heal has been established.

Example

A person living at home after spinal cord injury with a neurogenic bladder that has been suboptimally managed, as evidenced by incontinence and frequent urinary tract infections, should be considered physiologically unstable until appropriate assessments, interventions, and management strategies have been established.

Thus physiologic instability naturally implies that medical and physiologic conditions have not yet been completely assessed, diagnosed, and managed.

OUTCOME LEVEL I: PHYSIOLOGIC STABILITY

Outcome level I, physiologic stability, is the first and most basic clinical outcome level in the continuum of recovery and may be considered achieved when all medical and physiologic issues have been addressed and are in the process of being appropriately managed. Operationally, the achievement of the clinical outcome level of physiologic stability typically implies that the patient's major medical conditions have been appropriately diagnosed and resolved or stabilized to the extent that (1) discharge from an acute hospital (or equivalent) setting is clinically appropriate, and (2) all active residual clinical systems have appropriate medical management strategies established and in place.

The achievement of physiologic stability therefore implies that either all clinical systems impacted directly or indirectly by catastrophic injury or illness have recovered, or, if they have not fully recovered, appropriate strategies for monitoring, treatment, and management are fully developed. Typically, discharge from the acute care hospital setting to a less medically acute environment is appropriate, and intensive (e.g., daily) medical management and complex nursing procedures are no longer required.

Example

For a case of severe burn injury, achievement of physiologic stability would imply that débridement and skin coverage procedures have been completed, hemodynamic, respiratory, infectious, and metabolic complications have been resolved; and management strategies of sequelae are established. However, the burn patient may still require splinting and protective garments, and face future reconstructive surgical procedures.

Example

For a case of multiple long bone trauma, achievement of physiologic stability would imply that all acute fractures have been definitively diagnosed and stabilized and show evidence of healing without indication of other physiologic system complications. However, the patient may continue to require a cast with weight-bearing restrictions.

LEVEL I FACTORS INFLUENCING THE ACHIEVEMENT OF OUTCOME LEVELS II, III, IV, AND V

For the purposes of this discussion, we will assume that during the period of physiologic instability the provision of definitive care (e.g., diagnostic tests, fluid replacement, respiratory support, surgical interventions, monitoring, administration of antibiotics and other drugs) to resolve the physiologic instability and to achieve a level I outcome has begun and is in process. The perspective of global outcome assumes the necessity, in each catastrophic case, also to drive for and achieve outcome levels II, III, IV, and V, thereby mandating a further array of interventions and planning beyond simple achievement of medical and physiologic stability. (See Chapter 2 for further discussion of these levels.) An initial and ongoing appreciation of the need to achieve subsequent outcome levels reveals the need for the provision of additional services as part of outcome level I beyond those necessary for acute medical management. These services may include preventative rehabilitation evaluations and therapy identification of and referral to appropriate rehabilitation or other treatment programs or resources, and initiation of planning for future care needs. Even as acute management is occurring it is important to take steps to begin moving toward optimal solutions for maintenance of physiologic stability, for safe and appropriate discharge to a long-term setting (ideally return to home), for reintegration back into the community, and for return to work or school.

Patient-specific outcomes for level II (i.e., those necessary to assure physiologic maintenance) are typically achieved within acute rehabilitation centers. Some components of treatment to achieve this outcome level may also be provided in less acute settings. Outcome level II refers to moving a patient through all necessary management in order to discharge him or her safely to a long-term living setting (home, chronic care facility, etc.). Patient-specific goals relative to the physiologic maintenance clinical outcome are designed to accommodate each patient's needs and capacity.

Secondary Medical Complications

Secondary medical complications as a result of injury or illness, altered body systems, and medical interventions may significantly impact mortality and morbidity from catastrophic injury or illness. We will not recapitulate the multitude of potential secondary complications, which are more than adequately discussed elsewhere, but will illustrate the potential compounding effects on treatment and recovery.

Examples

The treatment of catastrophic injury and disease usually includes substantial bed rest and immobility. While such inactivity may be essential to the medical management of catastrophic loss, there are associated undesirable effects of immobility that themselves further compromise the recovery process. This so-called immobilization syndrome can develop when a patient is inactive for only a few days. The clinical manifestations of immobility affect almost all body systems and have the potential to cause secondary impairments that may prove to be even more disabling than that of the original injury. Clinical manifestations of the immobilization syndrome include (1) central nervous system dysfunction; (2) emotional and behavioral disturbances; (3) cognitive impairment; (4) neuromuscular impairments including weakness and deconditioning; (5) osteoporosis; (6) contractures; (7) cardiovascular effects including increased heart rate, decreased cardiac reserve, orthostatic hypotension, and thrombosis; (8) respiratory compromise; (9) anorexia; (10) constipation; and (11) compromise of other systems.

Depression may further complicate recovery from catastrophic loss. Multiple factors contribute to the risk for developing depression, including the organic effects of the injury or illness, the effects of immobilization syndrome, and the reaction to loss. The result of a complicating depression may be significant in the recovery and the ability of the patient to participate in treatment and rehabilitation. Failure to progress with recovery may further aggravate the depression.

Malnutrition is a major secondary complication of catastrophic injury or illness that potentially impairs recovery and limits participation in treatment strategies. Malnutrition is the result of inadequate intake to meet the increased caloric and nutritional demands of the response to injury, healing, and the recovery process. Inadequate nutrition may be a direct consequence of the injury or illness and required medical interventions. Anorexia due to injury or illness, immobilization syndrome, depression, reaction to loss, and the hospital environment may further potentiate malnutrition.

Identification of Individual and Support Resources

The achievement of levels II, III, and higher outcomes is optimized when the patient and/or family becomes a participant in the care and management process and learns how to assume active responsibility for the execution and maintenance of the necessary skills, strategies, and protocols established and taught by the treatment team. The sooner these issues are addressed in the course of treatment and recovery, the more responsibility patients and families are likely to assume for these results and the more potency or "leverage" the treatment team will have as instructors and leaders in this process. Therefore programs providing aggressive family education counseling and empowerment are essential elements of care in the acute setting (as well as in the rehabilitation setting).

Early identification of the resources and limitations of the patient and his or her family and support system impacts outcome planning and reverse engineering for establishing a treatment continuum. Psychosocial assessment provides an evaluation of the patient as an individual (including educational status, work status, relationship status, habits, and life style), together with his or her support system (usually the family) and resources, and is an essential component of long-term clinical outcome planning. The goal of rehabilitation should be to return patients to their own environment with a system in place that will maximize independent living, community access, and productivity, including the ability to problem solve to accommodate new limitations as the situation demands.

Other social factors may significantly affect clinical outcome and therefore need to be identified. Geography is clearly a factor in the availability and selection of rehabilitation services. Qualified rehabilitation centers and specialized treatment programs may not be located conveniently to patient's home and community, thus limiting or greatly inconveniencing family and/or support system involvement in the rehabilitation process. Legal factors are now, more than ever, impacting rehabilitation outcomes. Patient competency issues and conservatorships may affect access to treatment interventions. Patient resources, including contract inclusion/exclusions relative to third party payers, patient's status at time of accident (work related, home, third party liability legal status), personal resources, state and community resources, and disability, clearly impact the quality and quantity of rehabilitation services available. Third party liability suits with incentives for secondary gain may affect a patient's motivation for recovery, as has been substantially documented in the literature. State and local laws may direct or restrict treatment options and resource benefits. Now, more than ever, attorneys influence treatment in a broad variety of ways and therefore should be accommodated in the rehabilitation process.

Family Education and Empowerment

A common frustration rehabilitation professionals share is the unrealistic expectation of patients and their families that rehabilitation treatment will somehow cure their devastating losses. It is difficult to disappoint anyone who has such expectations. In addition, the patient and family often do not fully comprehend the impairments, disabilities, and handicaps that they face.

Example
The patient with a spinal cord injury and his or her family may clearly understand the limitations for walking, but may not appreciate the loss of bowel, bladder, and sensation functions.

Example
The person who has a brain injury may experience no apparent impairment related to movement or speech but have difficulty in relating to the environment, thinking, and behaving appropriately.

The role the family and the support system are able to play significantly impacts the outcome and durability of outcome in catastrophic loss. Therefore, the family and other support system need to be educated and empowered as early in the clinical course after the loss as possible. Even with a functional, supportive family, the impact of catastrophic loss may prove overwhelming. With catastrophic loss the individual and his or her family have lost control over domains of their lives that they had managed. The recognition of the emotional response to catastrophic loss by both patient and family, and its impact on their behavior and ability to participate in decision making and planning, is basic to effective education and empowerment.

The key to outcome durability is defining a reasonable global outcome and reverse engineering a plan that allows enough flexibility to accommodate the patient and family through the recovery and adjustment process. Identifying and evaluating appropriate levels of care and rehabilitation providers, and including the patient and family in the process, support is laid for effective decision making.

Example

D.D. is a 23-year-old man, status post severe closed head injury, secondary to a high speed motor vehicle accident. He has demonstrated no significant neurologic recovery over the 6 weeks since his injury. With the guidance of a case manager, the family visited an acute rehabilitation center, several subacute rehabilitation facilities, as well as a few extended care facilities. Although the family expresses great dedication to D.D. and would like to take him home, they have come to the agonizing decision that they are presently unable to care for D.D. adequately in the home environment. They decide to place him in a subacute rehabilitation facility that is about an hour from their home. Permission must be given to reevaluate the situation and make additional decisions as circumstances (including clinical status and resource availability) change.

The process of evaluating options is a normal process for human beings. It becomes rewarding when patients and their families become empowered enough to resume this life function by creating and analyzing options of their own. It is, therefore, important that the family and patient have permission to observe, explore options, make new decisions.

PLANNING FOR OUTCOME: EARLY STRATEGIES

The initial rehabilitation evaluation ideally occurs early after injury or illness, in the acute medical setting. Catastrophic loss often includes impairment and disability that broadly impact an individual's ability to recover, participate in rehabilitation treatment strategies, and return to the previous life style. The achievement of maximal recovery and independence depends upon the early recognition of all direct and secondary sequelae of the catastrophic loss. This evaluation allows for timely and appropriate medical and rehabilitation interventions to minimize the resulting impairment or disability, and handicap, thus maximizing the global outcome achieved.

By routinely considering, during the acute medical care phase, the subsequent need to achieve level II, III, and other outcomes, it will become apparent that early interventions must be put in place to minimize and/or initiate the earliest possible recovery from this secondary physical and psychological deterioration of the patient and family. Thus achievement of physiologic stability includes programs to provide (1) adequate and safe nutrition, (2) prevention of aspiration, (3) establishment and preservation of skin integrity, (4) maintenance of joint mobility, (5) initial management of bowel and bladder function, and (6) early mobilization (see Table 3–1). The clinical outcome of physiologic stability does not necessarily provide any significantly increased level of functional independence or restoration. Although varying amounts of functional restoration may be achieved in parallel with a process of achieving medical stabilization, such achievements are not an intrinsic part of the physiologic stability clinical outcome level. Treatment goals and strategies should set the stage for more effective definitive rehabilitation intervention in subsequent phases of care.

Table 3–1 Level I Patient-Specific Outcomes

Medical Stability	The resolution or stabilization of acute medical conditions and the establishment of medical management strategies to allow discharge from the acute care hospital. Specific acute medical issues may include: • multiple trauma • neurologic management • orthopedic management • spine stability • burn management • amputee management • respiratory insufficiency • cardiac insufficiency • vascular compromise • skin integrity
Immobilization Complications	Establishment of a treatment program to minimize the physiologic compromise and functional complications associated with immobilization and deconditioning.

continues

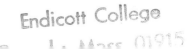

Table 3–1 continued

Acute Nursing Care	Establishment of clinically indicated nursing care routines and protocols to prevent secondary complications and allow for a safe discharge from acute care hospital, including: • wound care • bowel and bladder management • joint protection • skin management • airway management • feeding and nutritional program • pulmonary toilet
Nutrition	Establishment of a nutrition program that will maintain health and further recovery.
Preventative Rehabilitation	Establishment of a program for the maintenance of skin integrity, positioning, joint range of motion, and early mobilization.
Initial Rehabilitation Evaluation	Assessment of injuries, impairments, potential disabilities, and potential handicap. Outcome conceptualization and initial planning for continuum of care.
Individual Therapies for Basic Functions	As clinically indicated by patient's capacity, basic individual therapies for mobility, self-care, swallowing and communication.
Psychosocial Profile	Evaluation of the patient as an individual together with his or her support system (usually the family) and resources.
Realistic Goal Setting	Case conceptualization relative to projected sequelae of catastrophic loss, psychosocial profile, and available resources.
Analysis of Resources	Analysis of patient's abilities and comorbidities, support system, social, legal, and financial resources and limitations.
Determination of Appropriate Level of Care	Identification of appropriate and realistic discharge and future treatment options with consideration of the personal, family, health plan benefit and financial resources available.
Provider Selection	Identification of optimal provider with consideration of patient and family concerns, appropriate level of care, and available resources.
Continuum of Care Planning	Long-term outcome planning by case conceptualization that establishes an organized visualization of the rehabilitation process, including the identification of appropriate resources and options.
Family Issue Identification	Identification of family concerns and issues relative to catastrophic loss and handicap that may impact on long-term function and management.
Family and Patient Education	Education of the patient and family about injuries or illness, impairments, and disabilities, with the objective of providing them with a realistic understanding of prognosis, recovery process, and long-term care implications.
Family and Patient Empowerment	Facilitation of empowerment behaviors, including initiation, self-advocacy, problem solving, social networking, and productive activities.
Family and Patient Responsibility	Identification of the responsibilities of patient and family relative to the management of problems and issues related to catastrophic loss, including personal care, supervision and facilitation of appropriate treatment.

Clinical and functional assessments will define impairment and disability. Further, there is a large database of statistics available that correlate impairment and disability with clinical outcome. Great caution should be exercised in prognosticating clinical outcomes solely on the basis of statistical analysis of clinical and functional assessments. Clinical, functional, and psychosocial assessments provide the tools needed to determine realistic clinical goals and treatment strategies. Education of the patient and family relative to these tools can empower them to develop realistic expectations and goals.

CONCLUSION

Although these examples and interventions may seem obvious, multiple studies have clearly shown that routine attention to them can substantially reduce morbidity and resource utilization. This early rehabilitation planning is not only clinically efficacious, but also resource-wise. Yet it is also obvious that in the environment of acute care these interventions, which impact basically upon the longer-term outcome results, are routinely neglected.

Chapter 4

Acute Rehabilitation in an Outcome-Oriented Model

Ernest T. Bryant, PhD, ABCN

Objectives

- To provide the reader with an understanding of three primary factors central to acute rehabilitation; case management, team orientation, and setting of short-term goals to reach long-term outcomes.
- To define acute rehabilitation outcomes operationally for one diagnostic group.
- To present a model critical pathway for acute rehabilitation outcome achievement after traumatic brain injury and a critical pathway for the discipline of neuropsychology.
- To present a case example illustrating application of these principles and tools.

The purpose of this chapter is to provide the reader with an understanding of three primary issues that are central to an outcome-oriented approach to rehabilitation: (1) the value of a case management approach, (2) the value of a team orientation, and (3) the need to set short-term goals to reach long-term outcomes. The terms *outcome, objectives,* and *goals* are operationally defined as follows: an *outcome* is the ultimate result desired given a specific set of parameters (for example, independent functioning at home); an *objective* is a larger goal achieved, generally speaking, by reaching a set of smaller or more discrete goals (for example, independent ambulation, independence with all activities of daily living [ADLs]); a *goal* is a relatively narrowly defined result to be achieved within a short span of time (for example, independent ambulation for 50 meters, independence in oral/facial hygiene). The principles outlined here should be readily translatable into most rehabilitation programs and funding sources.

Researchers looking at rehabilitation program outcomes of patients who have sustained traumatic brain injury and other cerebral insults have generally examined five areas.

1. Changes in test or skill performance[1]
2. Successful return to employment[2]
3. Discharge living status[3]
4. Economic impact and/or costs of care[3, 4]
5. Changes in real life functional abilities[5]

Some of these studies used databases from post–acute-care programs,[2,3] whereas others have focused on acute rehabilitation care.[5] With the exception of those studies focused primarily on return to employment and/or with discharge living status,[2-4] in many studies the extent to which clear outcomes had been set at admission to the programs and whether those outcomes had guided the rehabilitation professionals in their program planning and in the determination of an appropriate length of stay (LOS) is unclear. Lack of clearly defined outcomes can unnecessarily increase LOS and thereby increase cost while effecting minimal improvement in an individual's degree of functional independence and quality of life.

In the acute rehabilitation setting, the desired "outcome" or "ultimate result" can be stated as follows:

1. The optimal use of the specified length of stay in order to
2. improve a patient's functional status across physical, cognitive, and activities-of-daily-living domains so that
3. the patient may be discharged to home with family support and, if needed, with a time limited day treatment or outpatient program designed to
4. increase the patient's independence further and facilitate the return to gainful employment, to school, or to vocational retraining.

Each of these four components must be appropriately addressed in a timely fashion with reasonable cost containment. Multiple barriers can arise, however, that interfere with goal attainment. Possible barriers include patients' becoming ill and being unable to participate in requisite therapies, potentially delaying their discharge; patients' plateauing part-way into their rehabilitation stay and not demonstrating further improvement, despite all efforts; family support's waning so that the discharge destination becomes problematic; and surrounding community programs' being inadequate to address vocational needs.

What, then, must occur if one is to optimize the potential for achieving the previously determined outcome while minimizing the impact of the many possible barriers? A central component of outcome-oriented acute rehabilitation is careful case management. Case management in the context of this chapter is defined as the careful monitoring of all aspects of the patient's medical status, progress in rehabilitation, and psychosocial issues so that interventions can be modified in a timely fashion to meet the patient's changing needs. It is commonly the responsibility of a specific rehabilitation team member but may be a shared responsibility depending upon the team's makeup (that is, a social service worker and a speech pathologist, or a neuropsychologist and a social service worker). A patient's functional status varies widely and can change rapidly. The ability to move a patient rapidly from one level of care to another or to adjust a given patient's individualized program to account for a sudden shift in ability requires constant review of the therapist's documentation as well as frequent observation of the patient. Continuously updated knowledge of the family support system and degree of involvement in the patient's care provides the staff with necessary input relative to the future caretaker's degree of anxiety, feelings of confidence, and actual level of skill. Such careful monitoring of all aspects of the patient's and family's functioning by the rehabilitation team can help minimize unnecessarily long stays in acute rehabilitation as well as in other levels of care.

In addition to careful ongoing case management, both the team approach to rehabilitation and a clearly delineated assessment of the patient's cognitive and functional strengths and weaknesses are essential if one is to achieve the stated goal in a timely fashion. Members of the rehabilitation team (that is, physical therapy, occupational therapy, speech therapy, nursing, social service, neuropsychology, and rehabilitation medicine) should set both therapy-specific goals as well as common goals, incorporating both cognitive and functional skills that all disciplines should address. The goals should build on the patient's strengths while attempting to remediate or compensate for the deficits. (For example, a male patient with an oral apraxia and right hemiplegia may also have some difficulty with attention and distractibility. The team can address the decreased attention by consistently refocusing him before initiating a given task. They can address the communication deficit by utilizing a communication board with pictures, letters, and words. Whether the apraxia itself would likely remit during an acute rehabilitation stay would need to be determined by the speech therapist and/or neuropsychologist. But what is most important is that the impact of the disabling "communication" problem has been minimized.) Such team goal setting and goal modification should occur formally at least once or more per week in order to account for the salient functional changes that are occurring. Team members need to view all therapy disciplines as equally valuable as their own. In addition, precisely because there are common goals, disciplines should expect that other therapists will frequently work individually and collaboratively on skills that appear to cross over into their own therapy's domain. Such cross-disciplinary collaboration *(cotreatment)* optimizes the potential for an integrated, efficient approach to rehabilitation.

The setting of goals and outcomes should begin before the patient's admission to acute rehabilitation. Once the patient has been admitted, these goals and outcomes need to be refined within the first 1 to 2 days after admission. On day of admission, the patient is evaluated primarily by the physician and the nursing staff, and if needed, by any of the individual therapists (for example, a speech therapist for an immediate swallowing evaluation, a physical therapist for specific transfer needs, or an occupational therapist for issues around feeding and/or hand splint management). Should the patient have a traumatic brain injury or complex cognitive or behavioral problems, the neuropsychologist should see the patient immediately upon admission to determine the patient's behavioral status and the behavior management techniques that may be needed, and to delineate motor, kinesthetic, visual, speech, attention, memory, and high-level reasoning skills. All of this material should be available to the rehabilitation team within 24 hours of admission. On day 2 or 3 after the admission, the patient's critical pathway should be formally initiated. Critical pathways are described in subsequent sections of this chapter.

All of the information, including the critical pathway data, is available to the case manager and the team. Throughout the first week the case manager organizes the team's input (including both the less formal "discussion" type of information as well as the more structured formal critical pathway data) and discusses the patient's status with the team. The team can then more intelligently choose the subsequent week's interventions to optimize recovery.

Setting goals and outcomes for acute rehabilitation actually begins before the patient's admission to the rehabilitation service. Physical therapy, occupational therapy, speech therapy, and medication management actually begin as early as admission to the intensive care unit (ICU), where individual therapists as well as rehabilitation medicine and neuropsychology staff evaluate and treat the patient. Even discharge planning from acute rehabilitation begins during the ICU stay. Social service or discharge planners should contact the family members to determine who will be responsible for the patient, what type of home environment the patient will have available to him or her, and the extent to which modifications in the home environment may be required before discharge can take place. Information gleaned at this early stage of care provides the rehabilitation team with some global parameters around which they can develop more specific goals within and across disciplines. For example, if it is known early in ICU treatment that a patient will not have a family member who can easily initiate transfers, the physical therapy department and the team as a whole can work with the patient either to minimize the difficulties in performing transfers or to encourage family members to search out alternative strategies for transfers should they find the physical demands excessive. These alternatives may take the form of using Hoyer lifts, having additional attendant care at specific times of day, and so on. In other words, all information that is relevant to the patient's current functional status, insofar as it pertains to the functional outcome desired, should be made available to the team for strategic planning.

In addition to the evaluations and the discharge planning, two other modes of intervention are useful in producing the desired outcome. The first of these, family involvement, is essential to both the well-being of the patient and the adequate training of the family to achieve the ultimate discharge destination: that is, the home environment. Family involvement, although beginning before admission to the acute rehabilitation setting, becomes more intense once the rehabilitation has been initiated. Family members should be encouraged to be present on a daily basis, if at all possible, and become actively involved in each of the therapy settings. At times, limits need to be set by the therapists upon the number of family members present and/or quality of involvement with the patient, but this generally can be negotiated through team meetings as well as through the social service department's interaction with the family members.

A second type of intervention is the cotherapy model, in which two different disciplines work jointly with a patient in order to improve the patient's cognitive and physical functioning simultaneously. For example, speech therapy and physical therapy staffs may work jointly in order to improve the patient's sustained attention and concentration as well as his or her physical endurance. The cotreatment may be done within a gymnasium setting while working on a gait class and carrying on a conversation with the patient or in a more complex setting such as in a grocery store, where the patient simultaneously has to walk, observe objects in aisles and on shelves, recall items to be purchased, and carry on a conversation with the therapists.

In order for outcome-oriented acute rehabilitation to be successful, interventions and the length of stay must be carefully organized and monitored. One method for establishing such a monitoring process is to institute critical pathways. A *critical pathway* is a systematically organized program that highlights those tasks that must be accomplished within a given time frame in order for the overall outcome to be achieved; that is, within each week, each discipline selects those outcomes that must be achieved for that specific week in order for the overall outcome to be achieved within the length of stay that has been designated. Each major rehabilitation diagnosis generally has its own critical pathway; for example, traumatic brain injury, paraplegia, quadriplegia, total hip replacement, and cerebral vascular accidents (CVAs) all have separate, individualized paths. Within the category of CVAs, there may even be more than one critical pathway, depending upon how a given rehabilitation center groups its CVA patients (simple CVA, CVAs with multiple medical problems, left versus right CVA, multiple infarctions, etc.). A recently developed critical pathway for traumatic brain injured patients who have an average length of stay of 21 to 26 days in the acute rehabilitation setting divides the critical pathway into three sections (see Figures 4–1 and 4–2): week 1, week 2, and combined weeks 3 and 4. Under

WEEK 1

Occupational Therapy	Yes	No	N/A		**Neuropsychology**	Yes	No	N/A
O.T. Evaluation Completed	☐ Yes	☐ No	☐ N/A		Neuropsychology Screening Exam	☐ Yes	☐ No	☐ N/A
Assess ADL's and Wheelchair Safety	☐ Yes	☐ No	☐ N/A		Assess Need for Psychotropic Medications	☐ Yes	☐ No	☐ N/A
Assess Cushion and Positioning	☐ Yes	☐ No	☐ N/A		ID Behavioral Problems	☐ Yes	☐ No	☐ N/A
Physical Therapy					Address Family Conflicts	☐ Yes	☐ No	☐ N/A
Bed Mobility/Positioning	☐ Yes	☐ No	☐ N/A		Assess Need for Acute Rehab	☐ Yes	☐ No	☐ N/A
Wheelchair Management	☐ Yes	☐ No	☐ N/A		Assess Post-Acute Rehab Needs	☐ Yes	☐ No	☐ N/A
Transfers	☐ Yes	☐ No	☐ N/A		**Speech Therapy**			
Gait	☐ Yes	☐ No	☐ N/A		S.T. Evaluation Completed	☐ Yes	☐ No	☐ N/A
Balance	☐ Yes	☐ No	☐ N/A		Assess Need for Hearing Screening	☐ Yes	☐ No	☐ N/A
U.E. Management	☐ Yes	☐ No	☐ N/A		Pt/Family Education Initiated	☐ Yes	☐ No	☐ N/A
Bulbar/Swallowing	☐ Yes	☐ No	☐ N/A		**Dysphagia ST/OT**			
Respiratory Status	☐ Yes	☐ No	☐ N/A		Clinical Evaluation Completed	☐ Yes	☐ No	☐ N/A
Documentation	☐ Yes	☐ No	☐ N/A		Swallow Precautions Posted As Indicated	☐ Yes	☐ No	☐ N/A
Recommendations to Team	☐ Yes	☐ No	☐ N/A		Assess Need for Modified Barium Swallow Study	☐ Yes	☐ No	☐ N/A
Nursing					**Community Outing PT/OT/ST**			
Nursing Evaluation Completed	☐ Yes	☐ No	☐ N/A		Assess Appropriateness of Community Outing	☐ Yes	☐ No	☐ N/A
Safety Issues Noted	☐ Yes	☐ No	☐ N/A		**Social Services**			
Environmental Controls Instituted	☐ Yes	☐ No	☐ N/A		Psychosocial Assessment	☐ Yes	☐ No	☐ N/A
Pt/Family Teaching Instituted	☐ Yes	☐ No	☐ N/A		Identify Discharge Plan	☐ Yes	☐ No	☐ N/A
Nutrition Collaboration with ST/OT/ Dietary re: Management PRN	☐ Yes	☐ No	☐ N/A		Refer to Rehab Family Group	☐ Yes	☐ No	☐ N/A
Affect Assessed	☐ Yes	☐ No	☐ N/A					

Figure 4–1 KFRC Critical Pathway/TBI. *Source:* Copyright ©1994, Kaiser Permanente Rehabilitation Center.

WEEK 2

Occupational Therapy

	Yes	No	N/A
Instruct in UE Programs	☐ Yes	☐ No	☐ N/A
Wheelchair Cushion & Positioning Evaluation Completed	☐ Yes	☐ No	☐ N/A
Family Training	☐ Yes	☐ No	☐ N/A
Dressing Self Care Progressing	☐ Yes	☐ No	☐ N/A
Need for Adaptive Equipment Assessed	☐ Yes	☐ No	☐ N/A
Homemaking Skills & Precautions Reviewed	☐ Yes	☐ No	☐ N/A

Physical Therapy

	Yes	No	N/A
D/C Goals	☐ Yes	☐ No	☐ N/A
Equipment	☐ Yes	☐ No	☐ N/A
Documentation	☐ Yes	☐ No	☐ N/A
Recommendations to Team	☐ Yes	☐ No	☐ N/A

Nursing

	Yes	No	N/A
Sleep/Rest Outcome/Eval Completed	☐ Yes	☐ No	☐ N/A
Family Coping Strategies Assessed	☐ Yes	☐ No	☐ N/A
Pt/Family Education/Training for CRL/FHA	☐ Yes	☐ No	☐ N/A
Weight Monitored/Assessed	☐ Yes	☐ No	☐ N/A
Behavior Modification Implemented	☐ Yes	☐ No	☐ N/A

Neuropsychology

	Yes	No	N/A
Assess Cognitive Status	☐ Yes	☐ No	☐ N/A
Assess Psychotropic Medication Need	☐ Yes	☐ No	☐ N/A
Assess Behavior Issues	☐ Yes	☐ No	☐ N/A
Address Family Concerns	☐ Yes	☐ No	☐ N/A
Assess Need for Continued Rehab	☐ Yes	☐ No	☐ N/A
Evaluate Post-Acute Rehab Needs	☐ Yes	☐ No	

Speech Therapy

	Yes	No	N/A
Assess Need for Augmentive Communication	☐ Yes	☐ No	☐ N/A
Assess Need for Memory Book	☐ Yes	☐ No	☐ N/A
Pt/Family Education and/or Training	☐ Yes	☐ No	☐ N/A

Dysphagia ST/OT

	Yes	No	N/A
Reassess Patient for Possible Diet Upgrade	☐ Yes	☐ No	☐ N/A
Assess Need for Modified Barium Swallow Study	☐ Yes	☐ No	☐ N/A

Community Outing PT/OT/ST

	Yes	No	N/A
Assess Appropriateness of Community Outing	☐ Yes	☐ No	☐ N/A

Social Services

	Yes	No	N/A
Evaluate for Family Conference	☐ Yes	☐ No	☐ N/A
E.H.H. Scheduled	☐ Yes	☐ No	☐ N/A
Family Training Scheduled	☐ Yes	☐ No	☐ N/A
Finalize D/C Plan	☐ Yes	☐ No	☐ N/A

Figure 4-1 continued

WEEKS 3–4

	Yes	No	N/A
Occupational Therapy			
Home Program	☐ Yes	☐ No	☐ N/A
D/C Recommendations Given	☐ Yes	☐ No	☐ N/A
D/C Evaluation	☐ Yes	☐ No	☐ N/A
Wheelchair Cushion & Adaptive Equipment Finalized	☐ Yes	☐ No	☐ N/A
Driving Recommendation/Limitations Reviewed	☐ Yes	☐ No	☐ N/A
Physical Therapy			
D/C Plan	☐ Yes	☐ No	☐ N/A
Home Program	☐ Yes	☐ No	☐ N/A
Family Training Day	☐ Yes	☐ No	☐ N/A
Documentation	☐ Yes	☐ No	☐ N/A
Recommendations to Team	☐ Yes	☐ No	☐ N/A
Nursing			
Family Training Finalized	☐ Yes	☐ No	☐ N/A
Discharge Medication Teaching Provided	☐ Yes	☐ No	☐ N/A
Home Care Instructions Provided	☐ Yes	☐ No	☐ N/A
Appropriate Supplies/Equipment Ordered	☐ Yes	☐ No	☐ N/A
Return Appointment Instructions Provided	☐ Yes	☐ No	☐ N/A
Neuropsychology			
Assess Vocational, Academic and/or I.E.P. Issues	☐ Yes	☐ No	☐ N/A
Assess Need for Psychotropic Medications at D/C	☐ Yes	☐ No	☐ N/A
If Needed, Family Training in Behavior Management for Home Setting	☐ Yes	☐ No	☐ N/A
Transition Family to Home Kaiser or Treatment Program	☐ Yes	☐ No	☐ N/A
Clarify D/C Plans with Team	☐ Yes	☐ No	☐ N/A
Transmit Cognitive/Behavioral Information to Post-Acute Program	☐ Yes	☐ No	☐ N/A
Speech Therapy			
Pt/Family Training	☐ Yes	☐ No	☐ N/A
Assess Need for Home Program	☐ Yes	☐ No	☐ N/A
D/C Recommendations Made	☐ Yes	☐ No	☐ N/A
D/C Summary Completed	☐ Yes	☐ No	☐ N/A
Dysphagia ST/OT			
Reassess Patient for Possible Diet Upgrade	☐ Yes	☐ No	☐ N/A
D/C Recommendations Made	☐ Yes	☐ No	☐ N/A
Community Outing PT/OT/ST			
Assess Appropriateness of Community Outing	☐ Yes	☐ No	☐ N/A
Social Services			
DME Order Submitted	☐ Yes	☐ No	☐ N/A
Post Acute Rehab Referral(s) Completed	☐ Yes	☐ No	☐ N/A
D/C Resource Guide	☐ Yes	☐ No	☐ N/A
Family Conference	☐ Yes	☐ No	☐ N/A

Figure 4–1 continued

PERFORMANCE AREA	DAY 1	DAY 2–3	DAY 4–7	WEEK 2	WEEK 3–4
Neuropsychology Screening Exam	Assess arousal, orientation (e.g., person, place, date, time), attention (e.g., sustained, divided, selective), sensory/motor (e.g., tactile discrimination, kinesthetic processing, grip strength, finger tapping speed), language (e.g., fluency, auditory and written comprehension, oral and written expression), memory (e.g., immediate and delayed short term recall of auditory and visual information, prospective memory, remote memory, source memory and new verbal and visual learning), visual spacial analysis (e.g., perception, integration), concept formation (e.g., similarities, differences), reasoning (e.g., inductive, deduction), control of affect (e.g., lability) and estimated intelligence. Determine Rancho Los Amigos Level.	Ongoing	Ongoing	Ongoing	Assess vocational, academic, and/or Pediatric I.E.P. issues.
Assess Need for Management of Affect or Behavior by Medication	Evaluate patient's ability to control affect or agitation via observation, review of records, and/or discussion with family. If potentially appropriate, discuss with physician and determine the type of psychotropic medication intervention needed.	Ongoing	Ongoing	Ongoing	Assess need for medication management of affects and/or behavior after discharge.

Figure 4-2 Critical Pathway—Neuropsychology. *Source:* Copyright ©1994, Kaiser Permanente Rehabilitation Center.

PERFORMANCE AREA	DAY 1	DAY 2–3	DAY 4–7	WEEK 2	WEEK 3–4
Identify Behavioral Problems	Determine whether patient is displaying inappropriate behaviors and, if so, what types of behaviors and their possible etiologies. If behaviors are inappropriate, set up appropriate intervention strategies for all staff to follow and notify staff of plan. If needed, write up plan and place it at nursing desk on unit.	Ongoing	Ongoing	Ongoing	If needed at discharge, instruct family in behavioral management strategies for in-home care.
Address Family Conflicts and/or Concerns		Confer with Social Services on family concerns. If needed, set up individual therapy session with family member(s) to address issues.	Ongoing	Ongoing	Provide closure with family and transition to staff at home Kaiser facility or at treatment program.
Assess Appropriateness for Continuation in Acute Rehab	Determine whether patient has sufficient goals to remain in acute rehab for at least the evaluation period.	If patient does not seem appropriate on initial exam, meet with team by Day 3 to determine rehab needs; if needed, initiate discharge procedures.	Ongoing	Ongoing	Clarify discharge plans with team.

Figure 4–2 continued

PERFORMANCE AREA	DAY 1	DAY 2–3	DAY 4–7	WEEK 2	WEEK 3 - 4
Determine Appropriateness of Day Treatment of Residential Services			Begin assessment of type of Post-acute treatment needed. Confer with Social Services on post-acute care issues.	Ongoing	Transmit necessary cognitive behavioral information to designated post-acute rehab program.

Figure 4–2 continued

week 1, each discipline has chosen those areas that it feels are essential if it is to provide a rapid and appropriate evaluation of the patient's functional status. For example:

- *Occupational therapy* must have a full evaluation of all cognitive skills completed by the end of week 1, as well as an assessment of activities of daily living (ADLs) and wheelchair safety, positioning, and cushion needs.

- *Physical therapy (PT)* will have assessed bed mobility and positioning, wheelchair management, transfers, gait, balance, upper extremity management, bulbar and swallow issues if appropriate, and respiratory status and must complete their documentation and have formal team goals and recommendations.

- *Nursing* fully evaluates safety issues, assesses the patient's affect, institutes environmental controls, initiates patient/family teaching, and collaborates on nutrition with the speech therapy, occupational therapy, and dietary staffs.

- *Neuropsychology* is to have completed a cognitive screening exam, an assessment of need for psychotropic medications, an identification of behavioral problems and family issues, and an assessment of the need for both acute and postacute rehabilitation.

- *Speech therapy,* by the end of the first week, has assessed speech production and comprehension and the need for a hearing screening as well as for patient/family education.

- *Speech therapy (ST) and occupational therapy (OT)* assess dysphagia through a clinical evaluation. They establish swallowing precautions as needed and determine the need for a modified barium swallow.

- *All three major disciplines (PT, OT, ST)* assess the appropriateness for community outings for the patient in that first week.

- *Social services* completes a full psychosocial assessment through interviews with the family and significant others, as well as identifying a discharge plan within that first week and referring the family to a rehabilitation family therapy group.

All of this information is tabulated on a critical pathway form and is available for review by the physician and team. Therefore, within 3 to 4 days of admission the specific information that is necessary for a focused intervention has been accumulated and is documented. By completion of day 7, there has been a reevaluation of the patient's appropri-

ateness for acute rehabilitation, an assessment of the need for appropriate medications, the development of a formal rehabilitation program, an
assessment of postacute needs, and an identified discharge plan and
ongoing family education across all disciplines has been initiated. A
clearly focused intervention plan is possible because the core elements
of an effective acute rehabilitation program have been clearly specified
and a critical path of treatment delineated.

Beginning in week 2, individual disciplines are now progressing with
family training, discharge planning, adaptive equipment assessments,
determination of the type of postacute rehabilitation that may be needed,
as well as assessment of the need for augmented communication, memory strategies, family conferences, and early home health evaluations. By
the end of the second week in the critical path, discharge plans are clearly established and specific goals of the rehabilitation program have been
carefully explained to the family members as well as to the patient.

Beginning week 3 and continuing into week 4, the primary objective is
to provide the patient and family with all the requisite therapeutic "tools"
needed to allow a smooth transition from the acute rehabilitation setting
to either postacute transitional living or home. Specifically, the rehabilitation team focuses upon finalizing equipment needs, completing family
training, developing a home care program, assessing vocational and academic needs, reevaluating the psychotropic medication needs, teaching
the family behavioral management techniques (if they have not already
learned those strategies), contacting the postacute care program (if
appropriate), submitting durable medical equipment orders, and developing a resource guide and a discharge family conference. In other words
the primary goal of the last 2 weeks is to prepare the family for the transition from the hospital setting into the home environment and to maximize the opportunity for a successful extension of the rehabilitation into
the home. It should be emphasized that while the critical pathway presented here consists of 3 to 4 weeks of intervention for traumatic brain
injury, other rehabilitation programs and diagnoses may have more or
less specific lengths of stay in acute rehabilitation. What is essential is
that the categories within the critical path are those core tasks that must
be accomplished within a specified week in order to achieve the outcome that one has initially set for the patient.

The goal of acute rehabilitation is to utilize the specified length of stay
optimally in order to improve the patient's functional status. Careful

management of the length of stay is becoming increasingly important in a time of fiscal constraints in medicine in general and in rehabilitation specifically. By setting outcomes early on, the patient, family, and rehabilitation team can all gear their interventions and plans toward achieving that specific goal. Such goal clarification reduces fragmentation of care and extension of interventions into areas that may have minimal functional significance for the patient. In the example presented previously, the patient, who had an oral apraxia, may not be able to recover functional speech in the course of her acute rehabilitation stay. To focus a speech therapy intervention primarily toward that end would be inconsistent with the overall outcome desired, which is to make the patient more functionally communicative in his or her home environment. The usage of critical pathways is one method by which the rehabilitation team can focus its intervention strategies to achieve the outcomes in an efficient and integrated fashion. Such a mode of operation is truly cost effective in that it minimizes ineffective interventions and optimally utilizes appropriate interventions in a timely fashion. In addition, an outcome-oriented approach allows the payer to measure whether the dollars expended have been utilized appropriately. Once one has established what the specific outcome is to be and has established a time frame within which that outcome will be achieved, it is easy to measure functionally whether the rehabilitation specialists have produced the outcome for which they have contracted.

The following case presentation is that of a patient with traumatic brain injury (TBI) treated within an acute rehabilitation program that uses an outcome-oriented approach. It is intended to highlight the factors that are most important for developing such a model. The primary desired outcome of his stay in acute rehabilitation was the safe discharge of the patient to his home with rapid return to an academic program and appropriate social contacts. This outcome was to be achieved within an estimated 3 to 4 weeks in the acute rehabilitation setting with possible follow-up outpatient therapies should they be needed. The frequency and duration of these therapies would be jointly determined by the rehabilitation and outpatient therapy teams.

The specific outcome chosen was partially influenced by the expected length of stay (LOS) and type of funding provided by the family's insurance coverage. Other funding sources and programs may have decided to choose a different outcome. For example, an acute rehabilitation program may have contracted with an insurance carrier to provide *all* rehabilitation programming at the acute level, and discharge would be predicated on the patient's ability to return to full schooling immediately without other outpatient services or extensive special education needs. Another option could be to keep him in acute medical care until it was medically safe to discharge him to his home, then provide a 24-hr/day in-home rehabilitation program with all therapies and behavior management strategies administered there. Both of these alternative models, and others as well, can still utilize the concepts of an outcome-oriented model to improve their efficiency and cost-effectiveness.

T.C. is an 11-year-old right-handed boy, who sustained a severe traumatic brain injury in a fall from a horse in the fall of 1994. An initial computed tomographic (CT) scan at the trauma center indicated a left parietal subdural hematoma with left ventricular effacement and basilar skull fracture. He had a Glasgow Coma Scale Score of 4 on admission to the emergency room. An intracranial pressure (ICP) monitor was inserted and yielded an opening pressure of 13. A repeat CT scan on day 2 indicated bipolar contusions. Four days post injury his condition was stabilized and he was transferred to the acute medical floor of the local hospital, where he was monitored by a pediatrician as well as a rehabilitation medicine specialist. Within the health maintenance organization (HMO) system that cared for T.C., it was possible to have the rehabilitation medicine specialist involved in his medical care and case management while he still resided in the regional trauma center, facilitating his rapid transfer back to his own medical facility and into the rehabilitation process. The patient remained at the acute medical facility for 12 days, progressing from a Rancho Los Amigos Level of Cognitive Functioning (RLCF)[6] III to RLCF IV by the 16th day post injury. Because this HMO program defines acute rehabilitation as encompassing RLCF levels IV, V, or VI, T.C. was then transferred immediately to the acute rehabilitation facility. From the time of admission to the trauma center and up to the day of admission to acute rehabilitation, the patient as well as the family were being carefully monitored directly by the rehabilitation medical specialist and indirectly by the rehabilitation neuropsychologist and the rehabilitation team social service worker. This early case management facilitated a rapid assessment of strengths and weaknesses and setting of goals and outcomes.

Sixteen days post injury, T.C. entered acute rehabilitation. On admission, the TBI team physician evaluated his physical status and determined him to be right hemiparetic with a nonfluent aphasia, impaired gag reflex, and severe agitation. The neuropsychologist also evaluated T.C. on admission and found that he could appropriately signal yes/no with hand signals, had intact visual perceptual skills, could read four-letter words accurately, and followed single-step commands with 80 percent accuracy. The neuropsychologist also indicated that T.C.'s agitation increased in the presence of bright lights and noise. On the basis of the physical, cognitive, and behavioral assessment, T.C. was placed in a quiet room with decreased lighting and in a bed with padded rails. Family and staff were to encourage him to use yes/no gestures. They were also told to speak softly and not to feed him orally until a formal swallowing evaluation was completed. The parents were interviewed on day of admission by the social service worker in order to introduce them to the rehabilitation department, assess his academic and social history, and begin discharge planning with the parents.

WEEK 1

On his second day in acute rehabilitation, all other disciplines began their evaluation of T.C.

- Occupational therapy completed a formal swallowing evaluation, together with an assessment of his ability to assist in activities of daily living (ADLs), his grip strength, and his coordinated complex upper extremity motor skills as well as his wheelchair needs.
- Physical therapy assessed his transfer skills, bed mobility, and active range of motion along with his wheelchair mobility.
- Speech therapy focused on assessing his potential for speech production, sustained attention, memory, and reasoning abilities.
- Nursing checked his safety and judgment while in bed, his continence, and his affect, while teaching the family how to assist in all of these nursing care activities.

Because of the complexity of some of these issues, assessment continued throughout days 2 through 5. By the fifth day after admission, formal goals were established by each discipline as well as across disciplines. The discharge plan was to his parent's home, where he would be provided with educational programming in that environment as well as ongoing speech therapy, occupational therapy, and physical therapy in an outpatient setting. Appointments for formal reevaluation by the rehabilitation team at 60 days after discharge as well as at 4 months and at 6 months post discharge were set. He would be followed medically by his local pediatrician. The neuropsychologist believed that appropriate behavior management could be taught to the parents so that there would be minimal difficulty in managing him in the home environment.

By the end of week 1, the *outcome, objectives,* and *goals* were specified for this case. The outcome and a sample of the objectives and goals are summarized in Exhibit 4–1. The critical path was also determined for this patient during week 1. The standard brain injury critical path developed by this HMO was deemed appropriate for this case.

Exhibit 4–1 Case Outcome, Objectives, and Goals

> **Outcome:** discharge to home with an academic program provided by the school district and with outpatient physical, occupational, and speech therapies as needed.
>
> **Objectives:** ambulation, functional independence in ADLs, improved communication ability, and increased short-term memory and reasoning.
>
> **Goals**
>   1. Have him reach out with his right hand.
>   2. Encourage hand gestures to communicate needs.
>   3. Reduce agitation by prevention of extraneous sensory input.

WEEK 2

At the beginning of the second week of acute rehabilitation, the patient and the parents were instructed in upper extremity range of motion and necessary splinting, as well as in wheelchair positioning. Dressing and self-care activities were continued and an assessment was made for adaptive equipment. Physical therapy determined what equipment he would be needing during his stay both in acute rehabilitation as well as at discharge to home. Nursing responsibilities continued with respect to evaluating his sleep/wake cycles, teaching the family coping strategies, as well as implementing the behavioral management program instituted by the neuropsychologist. The neuropsychologist determined that there was no need for psychotropic medication intervention as T.C.'s level of restlessness and agitation was beginning to subside. He did, however, spend time with the family addressing their concerns about ultimate recovery and their anxieties with respect to their son's future. Academic records were obtained and contacts were made with the school district to begin planning for his postacute educational needs. Recommendations on the frequency, type, and duration of PT, OT, or speech outpatient rehabilitation would be provided by those respective disciplines at discharge. The speech therapy department determined that T.C.'s speech was gradually beginning to return. He was changing from being aphonic to formulating actual speech sounds. Therefore, an attempt to move away from simple hand gestures to more vocalized yes/no responses was implemented. The team also felt that he would benefit from using a memory book since he was able to write. The dysphagia evaluation that had been initiated the previous week had indicated that he was capable of swallowing if provided an appropriate diet and careful monitoring. The family was instructed in the methods of feeding the patient, and under supervision of speech therapy and occupational therapy, they continued with their feeding program. The patient was being scheduled for a community outing for week 3 as he was becoming increasingly more functional and had actually progressed by the end of week two to an RLCF level V. During week 2, since social services felt that a family conference with all of the team members would be helpful for the family, a formal conference date was set. An early home health evaluation date was set (this evaluation would include having the patient and his family have an overnight pass in the patient's home, during which a physical therapist would visit and assess their equipment and safety needs). A formal family training day was planned for the third week. The goals established for week 2 on the critical pathway both maximized T.C.'s. potential for return home and gradually improved his cognitive and functional abilities so that he could return to the classroom environment.

WEEK 3

During week 3, each of the disciplines developed a home program that the family would initiate after discharge. Actual wheelchair design and appropriate cushion were ordered, a single-point cane was provided for improving gait, and family training in ongoing behavior management was continued. Return appointments and instructions on how to contact the local pediatrician were provided by the nursing and social services departments and durable medical equipment orders were submitted. A discharge resource guide was provided by social services to assist the family in contacting the appropriate head injury programs within their geographical area. Each discipline provided family training to individual family members in order to facilitate their understanding of what T.C. would need after discharge.

DISCHARGE

T.C. was discharged after a 26-day stay in acute rehabilitation. He returned to his home with his parents and a tutorial academic program was provided by the school district within 1 week of his discharge. He continued in that program for approximately 4 months before transferring into a regular classroom. During the course of that initial stay at home, T.C. received outpatient physical therapy to improve his gait, as well as speech therapy to continue his recovery of his speech functions. He was seen at 2 months post discharge by the neuropsychologist, who readministered several of the objective tests that had been originally administered during week 3 of his stay in acute rehabilitation. This information provided feedback to the school district and to the parents and patient as to the course of his recovery. His program was then adjusted to take into account his improvement across most cognitive skills and to incorporate other types of interventions for those areas that were still weak.

This case illustrates that from the time a patient enters the rehabilitation process, whether in the trauma center with comanagement by a rehabilitation medicine specialist or more specifically on admission to acute rehabilitation, all program efforts must be oriented specifically to the outcome that the rehabilitation team has established with the family. Once that outcome is clearly delineated and the length of stay has been firmly established, all objectives and goals from the respective disciplines are oriented toward maximizing the likelihood that the outcome will take place within the requisite length of time. Other rehabilitation interventions that may delay the achievement of the outcome are not implemented at that particular time. In the case of T.C., the primary outcome was to have him discharged to home when he could be appropriately managed. To delay his discharge to home in order to have him maximally ready for immediate entrance into the classroom setting or so that all gait and speech issues would have been resolved would have been inappropriate.

The goal of acute rehabilitation is to utilize a specified length of stay optimally in order to allow a patient to return to home and productivity with the requisite functional skills. For many patients, especially those with a mild to moderate CVA or TBI, a program at either acute rehabilitation only or a skilled nursing facility (SNF) followed by acute rehabilitation may be the only multidisciplinary rehabilitation programming required other than individual brief outpatient or home health physical therapy, occupational therapy, or speech therapy. Patients with such a mild to moderate degree of cerebral insult may need 3 weeks or less of SNF care followed by an intensive acute rehabilitation program before discharge to home. Family members can then follow through with the recommended home programs provided by the acute care staff. Once again, however, to return the patient to home and productive living within this relatively modest length of stay successfully, the outcome must be set at the very beginning of or before acute rehabilitation so that family, staff, and hospital/insurance reviewers are clear about what is to be accomplished and the specific time frame. Critical pathways can prove as useful here as with the more severely impaired patients. The following is a case illustration of a mild, rapid movement case.

S.G. was a 50-year-old right-handed woman with a master's degree in education who sustained a brain stem infarction secondary to mitrovalve surgery in early 1992. She demonstrated left-sided weakness and right hemiplegia, severe dysarthria, left ptosis, decreased proprioception on the right side, and ataxia. The patient was initially treated and stabilized in her local medical facility. After she was transferred from the emergency room to the medical floor, the discharge planning department at that facility notified the regional rehabilitation facility of her status and tracking of her progress by the regional rehabilitation facility was initiated. A rehabilitation nurse contacted her treating physician, therapists, and nurses once each week for 6 weeks and then determined she was ready for admission to acute rehabilitation. During those 6 weeks, the rehabilitation facility's social service worker contacted the patient's husband to discuss discharge planning upon completion of acute rehabilitation and to address any concerns he might have. An appointment was set for the husband to visit the rehabilitation facility and meet with the appropriate staff. At 51 days post infarction, S.G. was admitted for acute rehabilitation (this same tracking process would have been implemented at the SNF level had this patient been transferred from the acute hospital to a SNF rather than directly to acute rehabilitation).

WEEK 1

On day of admission, S.G. was evaluated by a rehabilitation medicine physician and found to have severe dysarthria, cognitive confusion, and a right hemiplegia with left-sided weakness. The social service worker met with the husband and sister to discuss the acute rehabilitation program, probable length of stay, anticipated postacute rehabilitation needs, and discharge planning in general. She also gathered information relative to educational background, career, living situation (carpeting, stairs, width of doorways, etc.), financial status of the couple, and "goals" that the family had set for her to achieve during her rehabilitation stay. The family was referred to a family support group and the patient was referred to a stroke support group, both of which were provided at the rehabilitation center. Nursing completed an initial assessment of the patient (critical path) including review of medications previously and presently ordered, prior diet orders, degree of extremity weakness, functional cognition, safety awareness, dysarthria, continence, pain, anxiety, and depression. Leg measurements were taken to assess for possible deep vein thrombosis (DVT). Nursing also explained her few dietary restrictions and safety considerations to the husband and sister. Since she was already continent, no new bowel or bladder program was necessary. A dysphagia evaluation had been done at the acute hospital and she was found to have a normal swallow and gag reflex with no aspiration. Safety precautions for cardiac concerns and falls (a posey vest) were initiated. Normal vital signs were recorded and paperwork was completed.

Within 24 hours after admission all of the disciplines had met with S.G., and within 5 days the team had initiated the standard CVA critical path. Occupational therapy assessed S.G.'s upper extremity management (ataxia, requiring slow, repetitive practice), evaluated her wheelchair cushion needs, and noted safety concerns (significant risk for falling because of ataxia and poor visual scanning). Speech therapy indicated that her dysarthria was quite severe and very likely would not significantly improve within the near future. Emphasis by all team members was to be on slowing her speech down, directing her to use a softer voice and to pronounce individual syllables. Staff were to reorient her at each change of therapy. Physical therapy checked her bed mobility, wheelchair management, transfers, gait, upper extremity function, and safety. Physical therapy requested that team members reinforce with her the steps necessary in doing safe transfers. By the end of week 1, a discharge plan was in place and the family was actively involved in the rehabilitation programming while also gaining psychological support. The *objectives* for her stay in acute rehabilitation were established.

1. Improve ambulation to a supervised or independent status
2. Develop functional communication strategies
3. Improve overall cognition and safety awareness to allow supervised to independent living in the home

Specific *goals* were also set.

1. Improve wheelchair mobility to supervised or independent functional levels (because of her ataxia and right hemiplegia, ambulation with an assistive device was not considered a reasonable goal in the 3- to 4-week stay)
2. Develop speech pacing strategies
3. Introduce memory compensatory strategies

With the team primarily focusing on these specifically functional objectives and goals, the outcome of discharge to home could be readily achieved within the 3- to 4-week length of stay.

WEEKS 2–4

Week 2 of S.G.'s stay in acute rehabilitation was again directed toward wheelchair mobility, speech pacing, and safety awareness. The team also chose to have her use a memory book to assist her in learning her rehabilitation strategies. Family education and training were emphasized in all therapies. Social service scheduled an early home health evaluation and finalized the discharge plan. In weeks 3 and 4, the therapies focused on completion of family training, development of home programs, finalizing of appropriate wheelchair and adaptive eating equipment, completion of discharge evaluation, ordering of durable medical equipment, and development of after care referrals.

DISCHARGE

S.G. had the necessary functional skills to achieve the desired outcome: discharge to home with few safety concerns and sufficient after care programs to optimize her overall recovery. Her acute rehabilitation length of stay totaled 26 days, while her home health therapies consisted of two visits each by physical therapy (for safety with gait in the home) and speech therapy (for appropriate implementation of the home program). Outpatient physical therapy was provided at her local medical facility to improve her gait and reduce her dependence on the wheelchair.

S.G. was seen by the rehabilitation team at 8 weeks post discharge. She was ambulating with a small based quad cane approximately 200 feet and was independent in her ADLs. She still had moderate to severe dysarthria and short-term memory impairment. Reasoning and problem solving, although they had improved to some degree, were still not at premorbid levels. As mentioned in the previous case history, while ambulation, clear articulation, and good cognitive skills may be "desirable" outcomes from an inpatient acute rehabilitation stay, they were *not* the outcomes established at the beginning of the rehabilitation program. Realistic functional outcomes in a specific LOS necessitate choosing a course of action that immediately addresses the more readily achievable goals while viewing more complex and difficult goals as long-term recovery issues.

CONCLUSION

This chapter provided guidelines for implementation of an outcome-oriented model in the acute rehabilitation setting. Actual lengths of stay, makeup of the rehabilitation team, as well as outcomes themselves vary across rehabilitation settings. Some specific replicable principles were identified to allow a more systematic approach to this area. This approach includes

1. setting clear outcomes before or at admission to acute rehabilitation,
2. determining treatment objectives,
3. specifying treatment goals.

After this process is completed, a critical path can be specified that will allow one to determine whether the goals, objectives, and ultimately the outcome can be completed within the time frame specified. This movement of rehabilitation into a more data-based, systematic, and replicable format will allow us to build on the strong clinical foundation that exists in rehabilitation and make the types of decisions on resource allocation that are going to be critical in health care today.

REFERENCES

1. Ruff RM, Marshal LF, Crouch J, et al. Predictors of outcome following severe head trauma: follow-up data from the traumatic Coma Data Bank. *Brain Injury.* 1993;7:101–111.

2. Wehman PH, Kreutzer JS, West MD, et al. Return to work for persons with traumatic brain injury: a supported employment approach. *Arch Phys Med Rehabil.* 1990;71:1047–1052.

3. Cope DN, Cole JR, Hall JM, Barkan H. Brain injury: analysis of outcome in a postacute rehabilitation system. Part 1: General analysis. *Brain Injury.* 1991;5:111–125.

4. Bryant ET, Sundance P, Hobbs A, Jenkins J, Rozance J. Managing costs and outcome of patients with traumatic brain injury in an HMO setting. *J Head Trauma Rehabil.* 1993;8(4):15–29.

5. Mills VM, Nesbeda T, Katz DI, Alexander MP. Outcomes for traumatically brain-injured patients following postacute rehabilitation programs. *Brain Injury.* 1992;6: 219–228.

6. Hagen C, Malkmus D, Durham P. *Rehabilitation of the Head Injured Adult: Comprehensive Physical Management.* Downey, Calif: Professional Staff Association of Rancho Los Amigos Hospital; 1979.

Chapter 5

Independence in the
Home and Community

Randall W. Evans, PhD, Leslie Small, MS, MEd,
and J. Scott Ling, PsyD

Objectives

- To present theoretical and operational practices for postacute rehabilitation in the community and home settings.
- To present a model that addresses the need for closer alignment between consumer and provider expectations in community and home-based rehabilitation.
- To present a client pathway and database for treatment planning, outcome projection, and progress documentation.
- To present quality assurance and quality improvement strategies associated with outcome-oriented rehabilitation service provision.

INTRODUCTION

In this chapter we present both theoretical underpinnings as well as operational practices designed to achieve the best clinical outcomes at the home and community levels. More specifically we focus upon rehabilitation services provided in community and home settings. The systems described reflect a decade of actual practice servicing a population of approximately 2,000 persons with acquired brain injury (ABI). While these practices have focused upon the group with ABI, the model described here can be applied to persons with other disabling conditions including developmental disabilities, mental health and nonneurologic conditions (cardiac rehabilitation). We refer to the "generic" client pathway to illustrate this point. Finally, the model described here embraces the need for consumer input and lessening of the distance that often exists between providers and consumers of neurorehabilitation services. We refer to "alignment of expectations" as a critical variable in achieving independence in the home and community.

THE GENERIC CLIENT PATHWAY

Clinical service delivery systems must contain well-defined and well-understood procedures that can efficiently enter/admit, serve/treat, and exit/discharge the target population. Ideally, a service delivery model should exist that could both in theory and in practice address the needs of *any* population. Such a model would not be theoretically constrained by time, by severity of the problem, or even by the resources available; rather it would be adaptable given variability in these factors. We refer to such a model as the *generic client pathway*,[1] as illustrated in Figure 5–1.

The generic client pathway is a model for outcome accomplishment. The model illustrates a set of actions to be managed by an accountable party (usually a clinical case manager) for each client. Pathway components include a dynamic clinical database, an accountable management party (e.g., case manager), and clinical professionals/paraprofessionals accepting accountability for achieving agreed upon outcomes. The generic client pathway allows for tracking of client outcome progression relative to the targeted goals and time frames for outcome accomplishment.

Upon entry/admission into the clinical program, assessment and evaluations occur in accordance with a standardized database used for all clients. Assessments and reporting of findings may either be comprehensive or focused, depending upon previous information available or customer request. The case manager then uses the database, together with historical data and data on the clients' personal, familial, social, community and environmental systems, and available sponsorship sources, to construct a *functional outcome projection*. This projection describes specific targets for intervention in living arrangement, needs satisfaction, productive activity, and identifies the resources and supports that will be required. Milestones that indicate significant movement toward the projected outcome are identified along the way.

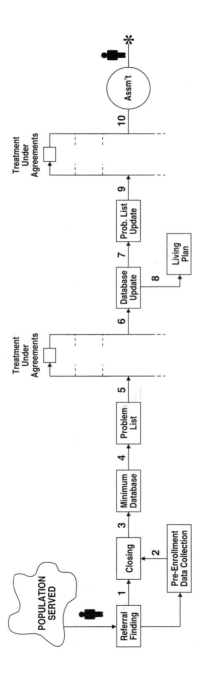

1 A referred client from the population served.

2 The required Pre-Enrollment Data set meets standards.

3 The client has been enrolled with required data.

4 The Minimum Database is complete to standard.

5 The initial prioritized Problem List is in hand.

6 Outcomes achieved as specified in Treatment Agreements.

7 Database has been updated (weekly) to reflect new findings and treatment progress.

8 Living Plan: approved by client, family, payer.

9 Problem List updated, reflects updated Database and Living Plan.

10 Outcomes achieved as specified in Treatment Agreements. Database has been updated (weekly) to reflect new findings and treatment progress.

Figure 5-1 A Schematic Representation of the Generic Client Pathway with Notation of Milestones at Which Audit of Client Progress Can Be Performed

Similarly, treatment is designed for goal achievement as the clinical case manager "contracts" for outcomes, *not* for services or disciplines. Once treatment begins, the clinical case manager and relevant outside parties including the sponsor and family monitor outcome progression to assure efficient movement toward the treatment end point. Check points, as specified in the treatment contracts, are used by the clinical case manager for monitoring reliability in meeting goals and time frames. For example, if the client is targeted for a return to work (RTW) outcome, check points include (1) completion of vocational evaluation, (2) job search, (3) employer contact, (4) job analysis, (5) trial work placement, (6) job acceptance, and (7) follow-up evaluation. The process is iterative: it is repeated until the client outcome is met. For additional detail on the generic client pathway the reader is referred to Wulff[1] and Jones and Evans.[2]

MINIMUM DATABASE

Establishing *the minimum database* (MDB) for any client, regardless of cause of disability or injury, is intended to be a basis for constructing treatment plans and functional outcome projections. The development of a "standardized" database assures that the treatment plan has an empirical basis. A database that is functional in and of itself defines the basis for client capacities, functional abilities, and resource descriptions of each client within the generic client pathway. The MDB allows identification of current client states that require change, effort, or services. Some components of the database will most likely have to be reassessed and reviewed continually, while others are less likely to change significantly or may change gradually. At a minimum, the database will describe the following client characteristics:

1. A description of the client's current physical, cognitive, and emotional state
2. A description of the client's current capacities and skills, which are updated at each iteration
3. A description of the client's prior status and abilities relative to characteristic #2

It is not our intent to advocate particular instruments, tests, surveys, or batteries that are most useful in rehabilitation. Some instruments favor different types of populations and the accountable clinical party or program decides which instrument best meets the specific client's needs.

The instrument must be considered valid, reliable, and relevant to the population under investigation.

After an extensive review of the neurorehabilitation literature,[3–16] the categories in Exhibit 5–1 were chosen for inclusion in the minimum database.

Exhibit 5–1 Categories for Minimum Database

I. Medical and Health Status
  A. *Physical Health*
    1. Physician's examination results
    2. Medical/health history
    3. Lab results
  B. *Dental Health*
  C. *Diet*
    1. Nutritional status
    2. Oral-motor functioning
    3. Allergies
  D. *Medications*
    1. Current medications
    2. Medication allergies
  E. *Health Risks*
    1. Seizure risk
    2. Other risks or issues

II. Psychological History and Resources
  A. *Personal History*
    1. Academic, military, and vocational
    2. Preinjury health status
    3. Preinjury living and need satisfaction status
  B. *Family System Adjustment*
    1. Current family makeup and dynamics
    2. Family education level
    3. Family knowledge of ABI and adjustment to injury
    4. Family expectations
  C. *Home and Community Resources*
    1. Description of the home environment
    2. Professional supports
    3. Traditional community supports (e.g., church, county extension services)
    4. Organized peer supports (e.g., AA)
  D. *Client's Social Network in Home and Community*
    1. Civic and other group involvement
    2. Network of friends and extended family
  E. *Financial Resources*
    1. Savings and other family assets
    2. Insurance and other sources of funding for services
    3. Entitlement programs in home community
    4. Legal status
    5. Earnings history and potential of client/family
    6. Financial resources required by client/family

III. Basic Functions
  A. *Sensory and Perceptual Functions*
    1. Vision
      a. acuity
      b. scanning
      c. perception
    2. Hearing
    3. Taste and smell
    4. Tactile Sensation
      a. temperature
      b. stereognosis
      c. light touch
      d. pain sensation
    5. Proprioception
  B. *Motor Functions*
    1. Strength, range of motion, and motor control
    2. Balance
      a. sitting
      b. standing
      c. during movement
    3. Posture
    4. Praxis

continues

Exhibit 5–1 continued

5. Coordination
C. *Functional Mobility*
1. Ambulation
2. Wheelchair mobility
3. Transfers
D. *Fitness and Endurance*
1. Cardiovascular conditioning
2. "Cognitive" endurance
E. *Cognitive and Learning Functions*
1. Attention
2. Information Processing
3. Memory
4. Orientation
5. Abstract reasoning
6. Learning strategies
F. *Executive Functions*
1. Goal setting
2. Problem solving
3. Initiation
4. Planning and execution
5. Generalized imitation
6. Self-monitoring
7. Self-directed behavior change
G. *Communicative Functions*
1. Receptive language
2. Expressive language
H. *Academic Skills*
1. Reading
2. Writing
3. Arithmetic
4. Study skills
5. Test-taking skills
I. *Social and Interpersonal Skills*
1. Negotiation skills
2. Conversation skills
    a. interactive communication
    b. turn taking
    c. topic maintenance
3. Assertiveness
4. Seeking of assistance
5. Giving of feedback
6. Receiving of feedback
7. Sexual and intimate behavior
8. Awareness of personal space
J. *Motivational Factors*
1. Reinforcer/interest inventory
2. Organic mediators of motivation
IV. Areas of Need Satisfaction
A. *Self-Care and Health Maintenance*

1. Bathing and hair care
2. Personal hygiene and grooming
3. Dressing and clothing care
4. Bowel and bladder functioning
5. Self-medication
6. Health management activities
7. Time awareness and punctuality
B. *Mental Health*
1. Counterproductive behavior
2. Psychiatric disorders (psychoses, personality disorders)
3. Personality factors and self-image
4. Management of emotions
5. Adjustment to disability
C. Nutritional Status
1. Eating and drinking
2. Meal planning
3. Meal preparation
4. Food-kitchen maintenance (oral motor functioning covered in section I.C.2)
D. *Housing and Household Maintenance*
1. Living space maintenance
2. Housekeeping and domestic chores
3. Ability to locate suitable housing
4. Safety-emergency awareness
E. *Accessing Community Resources*
1. Identifying and accessing community resources
2. Shopping for goods and services
3. Transportation
    a. way-finding
    b. use of public transportation
    c. driving
4. Community safety
5. Budgeting and money management
F. *Productive Activity*
1. Employment
    a. work skills
    b. work behavior
    c. work stamina
    d. job-finding skills
    e. job-maintenance skills
    f. employment potential
    g. job adaptations needed
2. Productive use of nonstructured time
    a. recreation
    b. leisure activities
3. Time management

As shown in the generic client pathway step 3, the minimum database, provides the basis for planning treatment, documenting milestones, and projecting outcomes. It is important to note that as each MDB category is being assessed, the evaluator consider how the client's functional ability relates to the projected outcome. For example, if the client is determined to have the capability for return to work, family support for that return to work option must also be assessed.

To deliver home and community-oriented outcomes, a case manager, or designee, is responsible for ensuring the timely development of the minimum database, for adding data to keep the database up to date, and for filing all data in a prescribed manner. In addition, accountability of data integrity is the responsibility of the case manager. The case manager is therefore accountable for assuring that persons collecting the data have relevant experience in doing so.[1]

HIERARCHY OF FUNCTIONAL OUTCOMES

Because the minimum database contains a wide range of measurements, and therefore a potential wide range of outcome, categories and a hierarchy for functional outcome accomplishments must be present (Table 5–1). It is imperative that all participants in the rehabilitation process embrace the hierarchical model and understand their contributions within that model for each client. In the following sections we describe the importance of conceptualizing outcomes within home and community resources and parameters.

Conceptualizing Functional Independence

The continuum of care for individuals who have experienced traumatic brain injuries, as an example, includes the extension of the rehabilitation process into transitional living or community and home environments. The purpose of home and community rehabilitation is to maximize functional independence. There is also a focus on compensating for skills that cannot be restored. Sachs[17] emphasizes this focus further by stating that "a transitional program for head injured adults provides a short term set of treatments that promotes evaluation and development of the clients' practical independence and psychological independence within a supervised residence that challenges the clients with daily living activities and adult responsibilities, and leads to re-entry into the community." (p 6)

The goal of community reentry is to assist clients through transdisciplinary training activities to attain their highest level of independent functioning in community-based living situations. Individuals who require home and community-based rehabilitation usually vary in their rate of recovery. Preinjury characteristics involving levels of education, intellect, work history, motivation, support systems, and community and financial resources also must be taken into consideration.[18] As Table 5–1 shows, varying levels of outcome are possible. For example, a client may achieve independence in the areas of domestic stability, safety awareness, and daily living status while remaining dependent in the areas of community access and work.

A useful paradigm that distinguishes acute (i.e., hospital-based) service delivery models from postacute models is that of the *skill acquisition* approach versus the *skill application* approach.[19] For example, "acquiring" the ability to ambulate may be a primary focus of physical therapy while the client is treated within the hospital. "Applying" that skill in the community—that is, crossing the street or pushing a stroller—may be a primary focus in the postacute treatment setting. Making this paradigm shift is a critical aspect of successful integration into the home and community environment.

The functional outcome model attempts to answer the basic questions:

1. Where is this individual going to live?
2. What supports are necessary to live?
3. How will this individual productively spend his or her time?

Delivering home and community rehabilitation outcomes involves an analysis of the activities necessary to contribute to the highest level of functional independence one can achieve in the following areas:

- activities of daily living
- safety awareness
- domestic stability
- work/education pursuits
- leisure life activities and
- community access

Table 5–1 presents these areas and functional outcome levels.

Table 5–1

Outcome	Functional Outcome Levels					
	I	II	III	IV	V	VI
Productive Focus	Independent Able to self-manage	Independent with structure Assistance with goal setting Independent with follow-through	Dependent External assistance for goal setting and for follow-through	Managed Requires institutional setting with direct management		
Work Status	Competitive full-time	Competitive part-time	Supported/Volunteer full-time	Supported/Volunteer part-time	Sheltered full-time	Sheltered part-time
Education Status	Preinjury independence	Consultative services	Resource assistance	Special education placement	Special/residential placement	
Leisure/Life Status	Independent Initiate/Participate	Initiate with assistance Independently participate	Assistance with initiation and participation	Requires assistance in structured program		
Community Access Status	Independent with cognitive and physical aspect in new/familiar situations	Independent and physical aspects in familiar situations. Needs assistance with new situations	Independent with physical aspects. Need assist to plan, initiate safely access in new/familiar situations	Independent plan initiate and safely access assistance with physical aspects in new/familiar situations	Assistance with cognitive and physical in new/familiar settings	

Table 5–1 continued

Outcome	Functional Outcome Levels					
	I	II	III	IV	V	VI
Living Situation	Independent residence in preinjury situation	Reliant on family assistance to meet some daily needs	Reliant on outside assistance to meet some daily needs	Supervised living and support for meeting advanced living needs	Supported living to provide support for meeting basic needs	Dependent living provides total support for meeting daily living and productive activity needs
Daily Living Status	Resume/maintain preinjury independence	Independent with self-care. Higher level tasks with assistance	Assistance with some self-care. Higher level tasks independently	Dependent on others to meet most daily living needs	Recognized immediate hazards in a supervised environment alerts for help	Dependent on external assistance for self-protection and safety awareness
Safety Awareness Status	Able to protect self in an open/unfamiliar environment	Recognizes hazards and communicates needs in open unfamiliar environment	Able to protect self against hazards in a supervised environment	Recognize potential hazards and communicates needs in a supervised environment		
Domestic Stability	Members of family system resume preinjury roles. Independently manage legal, financial, and family issues	Members of family system redefine role and response and independently manage legal, financial, and family issues	Members of family system redefine role and responsibilities and identify and utilize outside assistance to manage legal, financial, and family issues	Members of family system redefine role and responsibility. Will require ongoing outside assistance to manage legal, financial, and family issues		

Identification of levels of functional outcomes and a coordinated focus by the clinical team of skill application activities in crucial areas of goal attainment provide opportunities for the client to achieve maximum levels of independence and success. Fussey[20] states that functional tasks selected for treatment should allow patients the opportunity to achieve some independence and success even where they cannot perform the task independently. Functional retraining should aim to utilize the abilities of the client in a structured way so that the client, the family and the members of the treatment team can "see" the client's recovery (p 71). The interrelationships among domestic, social, emotional, and productive activities, and health and medical aspects, as represented by the levels of outcome, present a challenge to develop a comprehensive, integrated treatment model that provides a broad spectrum of treatment activities. The continuous review of functional status is an integral part of the treatment planning process.[1]

Managing Barriers to Attaining Functional Outcomes

While the generic client pathway and the minimum database approach can be applied to other clinical populations, the rehabilitation of traumatic brain injury presents some "natural" challenges to attaining functional outcomes for clients in the rehabilitation setting. For example, recovery from traumatic brain injury is usually a progressive process rather than a degenerative process. Kreutzer et al.[21] have suggested that development of community-based neurorehabilitation has been gradual for the following reasons:

1. Persons discharged from inpatient rehabilitation facilities rarely have life-threatening medical problems.
2. The deficits/problems of "discharged" rehabilitation patients may be subtle in comparison to the early medical and physical deficits/problems that are obvious in the inpatient rehabilitation facility.
3. Patients released from acute care may be able to walk, comprehend language, and speak, thereby masking more hidden deficits (i.e., memory, attention, problem solving).
4. The relative subtlety of problems and the absence of data indicating program cost-effectiveness contribute to lack of free access to funding.
5. Thus far, there are few cost-effective community service delivery models developed for persons with other types of disability that could be adapted for persons with brain injury.

Kreutzer and associates'[18] analysis, taken as a whole, demonstrates unique challenges for the home and community rehabilitation process. Overcoming these issues through the application of the MDB and the functional outcome model has been reliably demonstrated.[2] The traditional medical model of service delivery focuses on the attainment of individual and sometimes isolated skills. The acute medical model therefore places considerable responsibility on the families and other members of the client's external support system to integrate the individual skills into a comprehensive relearning program in which learning is applied to all aspects of the living situation.[22-25] However, acquiring and sustaining functional outcomes require the ability to integrate skills and apply learning in a broad spectrum of traditional clinical and functional areas.[3,6] While it must be recognized that family and community support personnel/systems ultimately must play pivotal roles in outcome durability and outcome application, this outcome-oriented, functional approach places accountability on the rehabilitation provider to make that transition effective.

TREATMENT PLANNING, EXECUTION, AND DOCUMENTATION

The fact that damage from brain injury is often manifested in many functional domains necessitates treatment intervention by therapists representing a spectrum of clinical disciplines who are capable of working as an integrated and complementary team. It is generally recognized that the chances of an optimal outcome are enhanced when the professionals who treat the client work in close cooperation.

The critical "pathways" in the transdisciplinary treatment model include the following:[18,26]

- The admission pathway
- The minimum database evaluation pathway
- The initial client profile and treatment planning pathway
- The discharge planning pathway

The cumulative evaluation and treatment planning process places the client at the center of the transdisciplinary treatment model with direct involvement in all aspects of the treatment process. Coordinated planning requires a fundamental set of information (e.g., MDB), possible outcome expectations (Table 5–1), and a clear understanding of the sequence of activities included in the overall treatment process (Table 5–2).

Table 5–2 Client Treatment Planning Process and Documentation

Steps	Activities
1. Preadmission Evaluation	1. Clinical evaluator assesses client prior to admission. Alignment of expectations with clinical needs. Provides current status from previous services/evaluations.
2. Preadmission Meeting	2. Clinical team reviews client status/expectations. Prioritizes clinical needs/activities; develops assessment time line.
3. Customer Expectations	3. Identification and alignment of client, family, payer expectations.
4. Complete Evaluation Activities	4. Priority evaluation activities to develop treatment plan.
5. Interdisciplinary Treatment Planning Formulation of Projected Discharge Plan	5. Clinical collaboration to develop treatment plan; the focus is on functional outcomes.
6. Client Participation	6. Treatment goals are developed in conjunction with client/family and provided to client in writing in the form of client participation forms.
7. Initial Client Profile	7. Comprehensive summary of evaluation results and individual treatment plan is developed. Functional outcomes and projected time lines are included.
8. Monthly Progress Reports	8. Written update of progress toward goal attainment is completed. Includes revised goals and time line adjustments.
9. Ongoing Refinement of Discharge Plan	9. Review of client status/progress/clinical needs in regularly scheduled case management meetings.
10. Discharge Summary/Graduation Report	10. Comprehensive summary of functional outcome status based upon completion of treatment goals.
11. Discharge	11. Successful completion/modification of treatment goals. Discharge status summarized by case manager.

A critical factor in the service delivery model for attaining maximum functional independence is also the client's investment in determining the goals and the direction of treatment.[27,28] The involvement and motivation of the client are considered fundamental to long-term success. Development of a minimum database of information is essential to comprehensive treatment planning and provides assurances that fundamental questions are answered during the development of the initial client profile (ICP). The ICP and accompanying problem list are primary tools in monitoring client outcome achievement. The ICP is used to *direct* movement of the client from attainment of one milestone to attainment of another until the projected outcome is complete. The ICP is the basis for identifying both basic rehabilitation and functional outcome goals and for achieving those goals. In addition, it provides an index by which interventions and client progression toward outcomes may be monitored and efficiently managed.[29]

The management of the client through critical pathways is achieved by gathering data and evaluation information and prioritizing the treatment goals. Clients "move" through the pathway, progressing from milestone to milestone. As indicated earlier, the generic client pathway (Figure 5–1) provides a model for outcome achievement in general. Individualized milestones leading to functional outcomes for individual clients are defined through the treatment planning process and are managed through the clinical case management system.

The development of individual treatment plans is a collaborative interdisciplinary process that relies on both the clinical expertise of individual clinicians and the effectiveness of the clinical team as a whole. Effectiveness issues can be measured vis-à-vis quality improvement mechanisms and thorough program evaluation.[30,31] Structure is provided to treatment planning discussions by focusing on the current functional status of the client and the projected functional outcome (Table 5–1), given an identified time frame for completion of the treatment program. The collaborative effort in developing transdisciplinary treatment plans contributes to the overall treatment milieu.[32] Monthly progress notes and discharge (graduation) summaries provide relevant parties with objective updates of treatment activities and outcome status.

MANAGEMENT OF TREATMENT SERVICES

Neurorehabilitation services, like other service delivery systems, face challenges of "risk management."[33] When rehabilitation is facility-based, as is the case with hospitals, there is a strong tendency to avoid "risky" situations for the patient. A simplistic example is that in most hospital settings most patients are transported via wheelchair at the time of discharge, regardless of their ambulatory status. A postacute approach could be considered to *embrace* risk by placing patients (clients) in more challenging and potentially riskier circumstances. In this regard, postacute programming offers unique challenges to risk management that are addressed in the discussion that follows.

Clinical and Risk Management

The postacute program is purposely designed to emphasize the community-integrated approach to acquired brain injury rehabilitation.[34] This design philosophy is apparent in the architecture, staffing configuration, program size, treatment venues, treatment goals and objectives, and treatment documentation.[3, 18, 32]

The goal of the professional staff is to develop and utilize an "applied" rehabilitation model in community settings as a means of achieving maximum outcomes for the clients. As stated earlier, "applied" rehabilitation is differentiated from traditional complementary rehabilitation by its emphasis on community-based skill application technology, not just skill restoration technology.[19] The professional staff share a common goal related to the ultimate measure of success in brain injury rehabilitation; applied rehabilitation results in the maximum emancipation from care and assistance so that the client can exercise independence and achieve maximum gain from opportunities in life.[35-37] The clinical treatment staff comprises licensed or certified clinical professionals; direct care staff are employed as specialists who are clinically assigned to, trained by, and supervised by licensed clinical staff; consulting physicians and services are available in the larger community. The hierarchical model (Table 5–1) is the focal point for all community and home rehabilitation outcomes.

The organizational structure of the clinical staff and the specialists provides an opportunity for treatment to be extended throughout the treatment milieu. Application of skills acquired in direct therapy sessions is extended, supervised, and practiced in all aspects of the residential setting. Transdisciplinary problem solving, goal setting, supervision, and extension of treatment permit continuous opportunities to evaluate progress and to maximize opportunities for success in increasing and sustaining functional independence (Table 5–1). For example, treatment professionals may elect to assess and train a client toward achieving a return to work outcome at his or her place of employment rather than rely on simulated tasks or environments. This training would include the vocational specialist and other therapists who have a direct impact on the return to work outcome.

The focus on outcomes provides a basis for identifying risk management strategies. Managing risk then becomes a part of the treatment planning process. Because the majority of postacute conditions carry little life-threatening risk, risk management focuses upon long-term issues such as the person's ability to return to preinjury life style behaviors (i.e., living independently, working, going to school, etc.). Therefore, a critical "risk" issue focuses upon "alignment of expectations," which is addressed in the following discussion.

Members of the clinical staff are expected to provide clinical activities that are in accordance with established program treatment policies and procedures and in a manner consistent with recognized standards of quality. The treatment professional frequently provides services in nontraditional settings (at work, school, recreational, or other community settings). Therefore, "specialists" (often bachelor's degree level staff) in specific clinical areas provide additional support and training to clients at nontraditional times (evenings; weekends). Some have referred to this as the "job coach" or "life coach" model of community integration.[19] The relationships of the clinical/specialist/management/support staff are collegial with individuals exercising the clinical prerogative to make recommendations that relate to their clinical and overall program functions.

ALIGNMENT OF EXPECTATIONS

Almost without exception, individuals who progress through stages of rehabilitation "transition" from one therapist to the next, from one facility to next, or from one program to the next.[20,38,39] This continuum approach, while beneficial to the recipient of services in many ways, carries an inherent risk of "misalignment" of outcome expectations. For example, clients and/or families commonly receive conflicting messages about client outcomes from health care professionals. A neurosurgeon's definition of a good outcome may not coincide with a neuropsychologist's. Therefore, it is important for the rehabilitation provider to determine the expectations of all parties involved (client, family, financial sponsor, etc.) as soon as possible.[40] Recent congressional hearings demonstrated that when the alignment issue is not addressed, poor customer satisfaction and compromised outcomes may result (*New York Times,* 1992). For example, at some facilities, prior to admission all participants are surveyed regarding expected outcomes. Where discrepancies occur, educational strategies and outcome check points are firmly established. This sharing of information brings the disparate parties more fully into alignment.

An example of the potential discrepancies between outcome priorities derived from postacute neurorehabilitation is presented in a survey of the various recipients of rehabilitation services (Table 5–3).[41] The Commission on Accreditation of Rehabilitation Facilities[42] requires that all CARF-accredited agencies have a policy on input for persons served. This is one way to ensure that the client or representative has had an opportunity to understand why particular services are being rendered and to have input into the rehabilitation process. Hosack's survey,[41] in which families and financial sponsors rank-ordered clinical and service outcomes (Table 5–3), indicated that while there was general agreement as to the desired clinical outcome between groups, "service" outcomes focus on clearly different priorities. Obviously, it is imperative to understand the priorities of the various consumer groups and to communicate information so as to supply each consumer with information considered important.

CONTINUOUS MEASUREMENT OF OUTCOMES

Outcome management is a dynamic process. The client's status is likely to change as a result of the combination of several variables including treatment/services, environmental manipulations, and variations in sponsorship status.[43] Therefore, at a minimum, it is recommended that the outcomes (Table 5–1) be continuously monitored through several stages. Several avenues are chosen so as to attend to the needs of the various consumers of

Table 5–3 Priority Rankings for Clinical and Service Outcomes

Clinical Outcomes (Equivalent)		Service Outcomes (Nonequivalent)	
Financial Sponsor Rankings (N=50)	Family Rankings (N=35)	Financial Sponsor Rankings (N=50)	Family Rankings (N=35)
1. Independence in activities of daily living	1. Independence in activities of daily living	1. Early identification of outcomes	1. Family involvement in decision making and planning
2. Improved living situation	2. Improved communication skills	2. Achievement of agreed upon outcomes	2. Training and experience of program staff
3. Improved communication skills	3. Improved physical mobility	3. Outcome durability	3. Sensitivity, respect, and caring from program staff
4. Improved health status	4. Problem behaviors controlled	4. Outcomes achieved at or below agreed upon cost	4. Intensity of daily treatment services
5. Improved physical mobility	5. Ability to manage own affairs	5. Outcomes achieved within agreed upon time frame	5. Outcomes achieved within agreed upon time frame
6. Client satisfaction with outcomes	6. Reduced need for supervision	6. Ancillary costs kept to a minimum	6. Family education, counseling, and support services
7. Ability to manage own affairs	7. Improved living situation	7. Forecasting of future medical and support costs	7. Financial sponsor involvement
8. Problem behaviors controlled	8. Improved health status	8. Client status follow-up after discharge	8. Availability of medical support services
9. Reduced need for supervision	9. Client satisfaction with outcomes	9. Predictable ancillary costs	9. Written progress/ status reports
10. Reduced need for rehabilitation	10. Reduced need for rehabilitation	10. Equitable treatment access for all persons in need	10. Access to other families
11. Improved employment status	11. Improved educational status		
12. Reduced need for health care services	12. Improved financial status		
13. Family satisfaction with outcomes	13. Improved employment status		
14. Improved financial status	14. Reduced need for health care services		
15. Improved educational status			

Source: Excerpted from Jones, M., and Evans, R. Rating of outcomes in postacute Rehabilitation for Acquired Brain Injury, *The Case Manager,* Vol. 2, No. 1, pp 44–47,[44] and from Hosack, K., Malkmus, D., and Evans, R., *Family Priorities in Post-Acute Rehabilitation for Persons with Acquired Brain Injury,* unpublished material adapted with permission from Learning Services Corporation, Londonderry, New Hampshire, 1991.

services, including clients, families, referral sources, and accreditation and sponsorship agencies. These avenues are likely to include

1. program evaluation[31]
2. outcome validation system[45]
3. continuous quality improvement, quality control[41]
4. quality assurance[46]
5. customer satisfaction[44,47]

Program Evaluation

The objective of a program evaluation (PE) system asks the question, Is the program accomplishing its objectives? A program evaluation system related to community and home models includes four key components: the minimum database (MDB), the outcome validation system (OVS), the analysis of customer satisfaction, and the quality council, which takes on special time-limited projects. The program evaluation system relies on gathering pertinent information at the beginning of the rehabilitation process that then drives the process. The Learning Services program evaluation system published in 1994[2] produces a semiannual report distributed to all staff members. Other outcome-related activities including quality assurance and continuous quality improvement complement the PE system; it is therefore both internally and externally driven. Internal activities include development of the MDB and OVS. External activities, defined as program responsiveness to input from outside sources, include satisfaction surveys and quality council activities.

Outcome Validation System

In the last decade, several "outcome systems" have emerged within the field of rehabilitation.[48] While our intent is not to advocate any particular system or set of specific outcome measures, we have attempted to coalesce parameters of outcome following comprehensive rehabilitation that transcends client diagnosis or cause of disability/injury, and to advocate a system in which all consumers can readily participate.

In 1991 we reported the initial findings of the outcome validation system (OVS). The components of this system were derived after comprehensive review of the medical rehabilitation literature, and objective surveys of a minimum of three consumer groups, clients and family members, referral and management agencies, and financial sponsors.[47] The authors of the study concluded that outcomes need to be reported in generic, broad-based formats so as to allow participation of all relevant members (Figure 5–2). In OVS, broad-based outcomes focus upon the person's ability: (1) to live at home (or a similar setting); (2) to live independently and (3) to be productive. The outcome validation system is described elsewhere.[40] This system has been included in over 1,600 consecutive cases managed within our system; it has become the foundation for program evaluation and continuous quality improvement programs.[42,49]

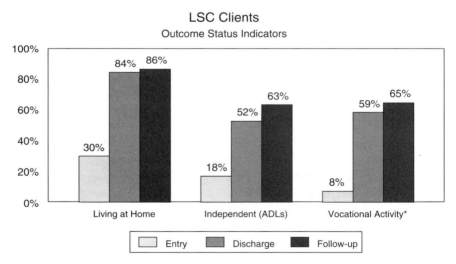

LSC Clients
Outcome Status Indicators

*Vocational Clients: Competitive: 6%, 42%, 49%; Noncompetitive: 2%, 17%, 16%.

Figure 5–2 Learning Services Outcome Validation System—Analysis of 1,623 Consecutive Cases

Continuous Quality Improvement

Continuous quality improvement (CQI) is an important component of the overall program evaluation system (Figure 5–3). CQI is designed to assist the rehabilitation team with monitoring the quality of services provided in each clinical area; to provide aggregate data; to meet the accreditation requirements of program accreditation agencies; to monitor the satisfaction of rehabilitation customers; to provide a mechanism for management and clinical disciplines to work collectively in the mission to uphold quality; and to provide an external monitor of quality outcomes. The CQI program at Learning Services utilizes a model that focuses on the interdisciplinary relationship between clinicians and management.[50] CQI is a component of the larger program evaluation paradigm (Figure 5–3). Like the MDB, CQI is an iterative process whereby clinical and management personnel receive ongoing feedback as to the effectiveness and efficacy of treatment.

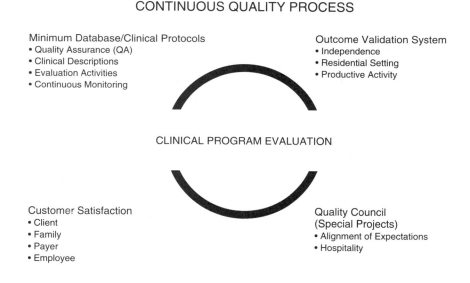

CONTINUOUS QUALITY PROCESS

Minimum Database/Clinical Protocols
• Quality Assurance (QA)
• Clinical Descriptions
• Evaluation Activities
• Continuous Monitoring

Outcome Validation System
• Independence
• Residential Setting
• Productive Activity

CLINICAL PROGRAM EVALUATION

Customer Satisfaction
• Client
• Family
• Payer
• Employee

Quality Council
(Special Projects)
• Alignment of Expectations
• Hospitality

Figure 5–3 Program Evaluation Paradigm

Discipline-specific "quality" is measured quarterly. Each clinical area is involved in training activities with a designated CQI coordinator. The coordinator assists with the development of quality plans and quality indicators. Actual clinical performance and processes utilized are reviewed on a quarterly basis by using established monitors, indicators, and thresholds for compliance.

The program objectives for the CQI protocol are to:

1. achieve successful completion of prescribed programs for each client served.
2. maximize functional outcomes achieved and maintained by each client served.
3. maximize value obtained for investment through optimal service effectiveness and efficiency.
4. achieve the least restrictive living environment for each client served.
5. maximize each client's independent living skills and minimize the need for assistance from others.
6. maximize each client's productive activity status.

The CQI program objectives are reviewed at admission for baseline assessment of functional outcome status and are incorporated into the individual treatment plan for each client; achievement and maintenance of projected outcomes are tracked through the outcome validation system (OVS).

Quality Assurance

Implementation of a quality assurance protocol provides for ongoing evaluation and corrective action as needed to ensure the quality of services delivered to individual clients. The purpose of instituting a formal protocol is to ensure that each client receives "high-quality" rehabilitation services.[51] Quality is defined with respect to the achievement of appropriate, functional outcomes at a reasonable cost. Formal quality assurance provides for case record review, as required by the Commission on Accreditation of Rehabilitation Facilities,[42] the Joint Commission on Accreditation of Healthcare Organizations,[49] and similar accreditation bodies.

For example, CARF program standards for *Assessment of Program Quality for Persons Served* are based on the following principle:

The organization should provide a mechanism for review... (which focuses) on the quality of the individual program of the person served. The review should provide an opportunity for suggesting needed changes. The assessment of program quality should not be confused with case records review (which looks solely at the content of case records) or program evaluation (which focuses on the aggregate outcomes of persons served). (p. 20-1.III.C)

To satisfy this program standard CARF[42] recommends a review process that includes the following features:

1. An established, written system that provides for internal review of the quality and appropriateness of the program of services.

2. A review process that includes professional or clinical staff and which may be performed either by an internal or external organization.

3. Quarterly reviews, including a representative sample of persons previously and currently served.

4. Management review of the results, at a minimum, annually.

5. Review should be part of the MIS, and used in program evaluation and market-based planning. (p 19-1.III.B)

Additionally, CARF recommends that the organization's internal review answer the following questions:

1. Are services initiated at the *appropriate point* during the person's program?

2. Were appropriate services provided for an *adequate duration*?

3. Were *appropriate goals stated* for each service in the person's program?

4. Did services *produce the desired results* in terms of the stated goals of the person's program? (p 20-1.III.C)

All of these issues should be addressed in the postacute provider's ability to meet its objectives.

Overview of QA Protocol

We have established a comprehensive internal review system for quality assurance. Included are clinical case management and quality assurance of the clinical documentation. The review is performed by an established QA committee that consists of representatives of the management, case management, clinical services, and direct care staff.

Each client is assigned a clinical case manager upon enrollment. The case manager is responsible for coordinating the client's treatment program and for monitoring progress to ensure achievement of acceptable clinical outcomes and judicious use of the client's financial resources. The case management system involves essentially continuous review of program quality. This ongoing review is documented in the client-oriented record (COR),[52] which is established and maintained for each client by the clinical case manager.

The QA committee provides an internal program review by a committee consisting of clinical and management staff who meet quarterly to review a sample of individualized client programs. The QA review involves an examination of the client's COR and interviews with clinicians and clients, as needed, in order to complete an evaluation protocol. Results of the QA review are disseminated to relevant clinical and management staff for review and corrective actions, if needed.

The COR review summary data are consolidated in an annual program evaluation report that presents findings from the outcome validation system with respect to client outcomes, from customer satisfaction surveys, from case record reviews, and from the clinical quality improvement data compiled during the gathering of the minimum database.

CUSTOMER SATISFACTION

Much has recently been written on the need to measure the satisfaction levels of recipients of health care services in the United States.[27, 44, 53, 54–57] As was illustrated in a recent issue of the *Journal of Head Trauma Rehabilitation* (1992) the perceived value of rehabilitation services takes on several perspectives. For example, as illustrated in Figures 5–4 and 5–5, there is rarely a perfect correlation between satisfaction levels and perceived value, particularly with payer sources.

Of significance was the finding that a "good or acceptable outcome" does not always translate into perceived value. Figures 5–4 and 5–5 suggest that the rehabilitation industry must do a better job at explaining or demonstrating the cost-effectiveness or "payback" of rehabilitation investments. It is likely that if the financial sponsor perceives a return on investment then the value of the service will be enhanced. The scores from these various satisfaction measures are integrated into the overall quality program (Figure 5–3).

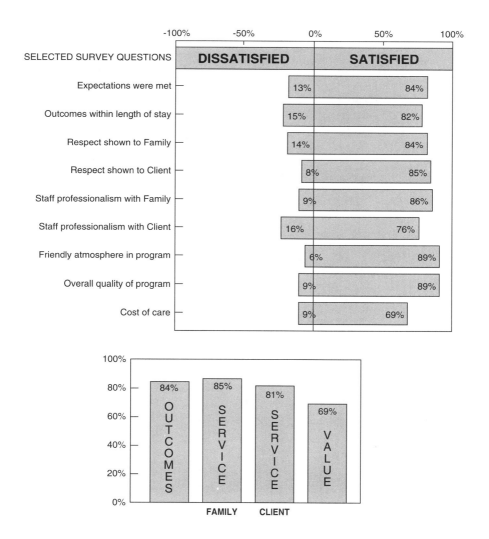

Figure 5–4 Client and Family Satisfaction Scores

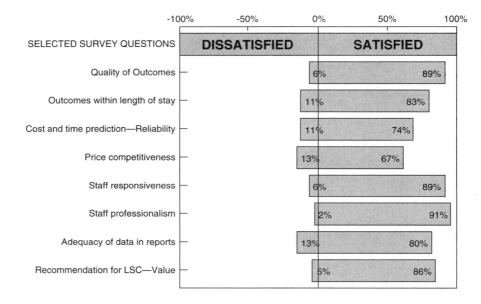

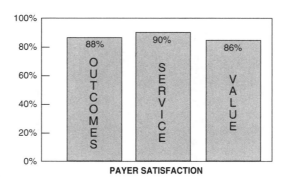

Figure 5–5 Financial Provider Satisfaction Scores

CONCLUSION

In this chapter we have attempted to demonstrate processes that lead to documentable enhancements of clients' functional outcomes. Additionally, procedures have been established whereby consumers of rehabilitation services have the opportunity to rank outcomes in terms of their own satisfaction levels and to determine the value of services rendered. The models of care detailed in this chapter could certainly be extended to other levels of health care practice. The fundamental issues outlined in this chapter, assessing the needs of the population served, including measurements that assess that need, evaluating the change in client's status when services are rendered, and determining the satisfaction level of consumer groups after service delivery, can be applied to other health care environments.

Health care practice in America is clearly moving toward an accountable model whereby the recipients of health care have greater input in the care process. We embrace such a model and have assigned our home and community rehabilitation model to support such accountable health care reform.

REFERENCES

1. Wulff JJ. Case management practices. In: McMahon BT, Evans RW, eds. *The Shortest Distance: The Pursuit of Independence for Persons with Acquired Brain Injury.* PMD Publishers Group, Inc; 1994:131–142.

2. Jones ML, Evans RW. Outcome validation strategies. In: McMahon BT, Evans RW, eds. *The Shortest Distance: The Pursuit of Independence for Persons with Acquired Brain Injury,* PMD Publishers and Group, Inc; 1994:73–100.

3. Boake C. Transitional living centers in head injury rehabilitation. In: Kreutzer, JS, Wehman P, eds. *Community Integration Following Traumatic Brain Injury.*

4. Dahmer ER, Shilling MA, Hamilton BR, et al: A model systems database for traumatic brain injury. *J Head Trauma Rehabil.* 1993;8(2):12–25.

5. Fryer LJ, Haffey WJ. Cognitive rehabilitation and community readaptation: outcomes from two program models. *J Head Trauma Rehabil.* 1987;2(3): 51–63.

6. Evans RW, Preston BK. Day rehabilitation programming: a theoretical model. In: Kreutzer JS, Wheman P, eds. *Community Integration Following Traumatic Brain Injury.*

7. Cope DN, Cole JR, Hall KM, Barkan H. (1991) Brain injury: analysis of outcome in a post-acute rehabilitation system. Part 1: general analysis. *Brain Injury.* 1991;5:111–125.

8. Gordon WA, Mann N, Willer B. Demographic and social characteristics of the traumatic brain injury model system database. *J Head Trauma Rehabil.* 1993;8(2):26–33.

9. Hall KM, Hamilton BB, Gordon WA, and Zasler ND. Characteristics and comparisons of functional assessment indices: disability rating scale, functional independence measure and functional assessment measure. *J Head Trauma Rehabil.* 1993;8(2):60–74.

10. Willer B, Rosenthal M, Kreutzer JS, Gordon WA, Rempel R. Assessment of community integration following rehabilitation for traumatic brain injury. *J Head Trauma Rehabil.* 1993;8(2):75–87.

11. ACRM White Paper. Addressing the post-rehabilitation health care needs of persons with disabilities. *Arch Phys Med Rehabil.* 1993;74:58–514.

12. Alfano DP, Neilson PM, Fink MP. Long term psychosocial adjustment following head or spinal cord injury. *Neuropsychiatry Neuropsychology Behav Neurol.* 1993;6(2):117–125.

13. Bach-y-Rita P. Recovery from brain damage. *J Neurol Rehabil.* 1992;6(4):191–199.

14. Brown DSO, Nell V. Recovery from diffuse traumatic brain injury in Johannesburg: a concurrent prospective study. *Arch Phys Med Rehabil.* 1992;73:758–770.

15. Kaplan CP, Corrigan JD. The relationship between cognition and functional independence in adults with traumatic brain injury. *Arch Phys Med Rehabil.* 1994;75:643–650.

16. Johnston MV, Hall KM. Outcomes evaluation in TBI rehabilitation. Part 1: overview and system principles. *Arch of Phys Med Rehabil.* 1994;75:SC-2–SC-9.

17. Sachs PR. A family guide to evaluating transitional living programs for head injured adults. *Cognit Rehabil.* 1986;4(6):6–9.

18. Kruetzer JS, Wehman P. *Community Integration following Traumatic Brain Injury.* Baltimore: Paul H. Brookes Publishing Co; 1990.

19. Jones ML, Patrick P, Evans RW, Wulff J. The life coach model of community re-entry. In: McMahon BT, Shaw LR, eds. *Work Worth Doing: Advance in Brain Injury Rehabilitation.* Paul M. Deutsch Press, Inc; 1991:229–302.

20. Fussey I, Gordon MG, (eds.) *Rehabilitation of the Severely Brain Injured Adult: A Practical Approach.* London: Croom-Helm; 1988.

21. Kreutzer JS, Leininger BE, Harris JA. In: Kreutzer JS, Wehman P, eds. *Community Integration Following Traumatic Brain Injury.* Baltimore: Paul H. Brooke Publishing Co;1990.

22. Alexander M. Acquired disabilities: new directions. *Dev Med Child Neurol.* 1993;35:753–754.

23. Brooks N, Campsie L, Symington C, Beattie A, McKinlay W. The effects of severe head injury on patient and relative within seven years of injury. *J Head Trauma Rehabil.* 1987;2(3):1–13.

24. Dikmen S, Machamer SJ, Temkin N. Psychosocial outcome in patients with moderate to severe head injury: two year follow-up. *Brain Injury.* 1993;7(2):113–124.

25. Wagner MT, Williams JM, Long CJ. The role of social networks in recovery from head trauma. *Int J Clin Neuropsychol.* 1990;12 (3-4):131–137.

26. Preston B, Ulicny G, Evans R. Vocational placement outcomes using a transitional job coaching model with persons with severe acquired brain injury. *Rehabil Counsel Bull.* 1992;35(4):230–239.

27. Condeluci A, Ferris LL, Bogdan A. Outcome and value: the survivor perspective. *J Head Trauma Rehabil.* 1992;7(4):37–45.

28. Melamid S, Groswasser Z, Stern MJ. Acceptance of disability, work involvement and subjective rehabilitation status of traumatic brain-injured (TBI) patients. *Brain Injury.* 1992;6(3):233–243.

29. Malkmus DD, Johnson P. Dedicated management of outcome, quality, and value: internal case management. *J Head Trauma Rehabil.* 1992;7(4):57–67.

30. Ashley MJ, Krych DK, Lehr RP. Cost/benefit analysis for post-acute rehabilitation of the traumatically brain-injured patient. *J Insur Med.* 1990;22(2):156–161.

31. Johnston MV, Wilkerson DL. Program evaluation and quality improvement systems in brain injury rehabilitation. *J Head Trauma Rehabil.* 1992;7(4):68–82.

32. England B. (1989). The rehabilitation environment. In: England B, Glass RM, Patterson CH, eds. *Quality Rehabilitation: Results Oriented Patient Care,* Chicago: American Hospital Publishing, Inc; 1989;11–18.

33. Carlson JG. Risk Management: Clinical and Financial. In: McMahon BT, Evans RW, eds. *The Shortest Distance: The Pursuit of Independence for Persons with Acquired Brain Injury.* PMD Publishers Group, Inc; 1994:43–56.

34. Shue K. Programma development: repatriation community programs. Part I: a collaboration model of service delivery. *Brain Injury.* 1993;7(4):367–376.

35. Willer BS, Guastaferro JR, Zankiw I, Duran R. Rehabilitation and functional assessment in residential programs for individuals with disabilities. In: Jacobson JW, Burchard SN, Carling PJ, eds. *Clinical Services, Social Adjustment and Work Life in Community Living.* Baltimore: Johns Hopkins University Press; 1990.

36. Ylvisaker M, Gobble EMR. *Community Re-Entry for Head Injured Adults.* Boston: College-Hill Press; 1987.

37. Ylvisaker M. *Head Injury Rehabilitation: Children and Adolescents,* San Diego: College Hill Press; 1985.

38. Whitlock JA. Functional outcome of low-level traumatically brain injured admitted to an acute rehabilitation programma. *Brain Injury.* 1992;6(5):447–459.

39. Long WB, Sacco WJ, Coombes SS, Copes WS, Bullock A, Melville JK. Determining normative standards for functional independence measure transitions in rehabilitation. *Arch Phys Med Rehabil.* 1994;75:144.

40. Jones ML, Evans RW. Outcome validation in post-acute rehabilitation trends and correlates in treatment and outcome. *J Insur Med.* 1992;24(3):186–192.

41. Hosack K, Malkmus D, Evans RW. *Family Priorities in Post-Acute Rehabilitation for Persons with Acquired Brain Injury.* Londonderry, NH: Learning Services Corporation; 1991.

42. Commission on Accreditation of Rehabilitation Facilities. *Standards Manual for Organizations Serving People with Disabilities.* Tucson, Ariz: Commission on Accreditation of Rehabilitation Facilities; 1994.

43. Valentine JH. Health Care Administration and Outcomes Management. *J Health Hum Resour Adm.* Fall 1993: 217–230.

44. Jones ML, Evans RW. Rating outcomes in post-acute rehabilitation of acquired brain injury. *Case Manager.* January-March 1991:44–47.

45. Evans RW, Ruff RM. Outcome and value: a perspective in rehabilitation outcomes achieved in acquired brain injury. *J Head Trauma Rehabil.* 1992;7(4):24–36.

46. Frey WR. Quality management: protecting and enhancing quality in brain injury rehabilitation. *J Head Trauma Rehabil.* 1992;7(4):1–10.

47. Papastrat LA. Outcome and value following brain injury: a financial providers' perspective. *J Head Trauma Rehabil.* 1992;7(4):11–23.

48. DiDonato BA, Schaffer VL. The importance of outcome data in brain injury rehabilitation. *Rehabil Nurs.* 1994;19(4):219–228.

49. Joint Commission. *Accreditation Manual for Mental Health, Chemical Dependency, and Mental Retardation/Developmental Disabilities Services.* Joint Commission on Accreditation of Healthcare Organizations; 1993.

50. Slater CA, Evans RW, Small L. Clinical program evaluation: an example of continuous quality. Presented at the Annual American Speech and Hearing Association Symposium in Anaheim, Calif.

51. Gray CS, Swope MG. (1989). Integrated program evaluation and quality. In: England B, Glass RM, Patterson CH. eds. *Quality Rehabilitation: Results Oriented Patient Care,* Chicago: American Hospital Publishing, Inc; 1989.

52. *Learning Services Treatment Operations Policy and Procedures Manual.* Londonderry, NH: Learning Services Corporation; 1991.

53. Batavia AI. Assessing the function of functional assessment: a consumer perspective. *Disabil Rehabil.* 1992;14(3):156–160.

54. Knafl K, Breitmayer B, Gallo A, Zoeller L. Parents' views of health care providers: an exploration of the components of a positive working relationship. *Community Health Care.* 1992;21(2):90–96.

55. Evans RW, Jones ML. Integrating outcomes value and quality: an outcome validation system for post-acute rehabilitation programs. *J Insur Med.* 1991;23(3):192–196.

56. Frattali CM. Perspectives on functional assessment: its use for policy making. *Disabil Rehabil.* 1993;15(1):1–9.

57. Wood RL, Eames P, eds. *Models of Brain Injury Rehabilitation.* Baltimore: The Johns Hopkins University Press; 1989.

Chapter 6

Outcome-Oriented Subacute Rehabilitation

William J. Haffey, PhD, Laura E. Cayce, PT, MHA,
and Louis E. Hallman, III

Objectives

- To distinguish the subacute level of care in the context of medical rehabilitation.
- To address the pragmatic realities associated with providing skilled nursing facility (SNF)–based outcome-focused medical rehabilitation.
- To address the substantial information technology needs associated with SNF–based outcome-focused rehabilitation.

Outcome-oriented rehabilitation seeks to produce the greatest value for consumers and purchasers of care. An outcome-oriented perspective defines rehabilitation's value as a function of the clinical results produced (disability and handicap reduction) and the price to the purchaser. For a given clinical population, value is enhanced by

- producing a greater degree of functional recovery for a similar price (greater effectiveness),
- producing a similar degree of functional recovery for a lower price (greater efficiency).

This chapter focuses on the pragmatic realities associated with providing outcome-focused subacute medical rehabilitation in a skilled nursing facility (SNF).

EMERGENCE OF SUBACUTE REHABILITATION

Subacute medical rehabilitation first emerged as a *level of care* for those persons with disability who were deemed ineligible for acute medical rehabilitation, either prior to or during an acute rehabilitation stay, for one of a number of reasons, including (1) inability to participate in at least 3 hours a day of multidisciplinary rehabilitation services; (2) lack of a need for intensive multidisciplinary rehabilitation, despite their need for inpatient care of mediconursing needs; (3) expected or observed rate of progress too slow or a magnitude of change too small to justify placement (or continued stay) in an acute medical rehabilitation setting; or (4) judgment that despite the continued benefits of rehabilitation services, the patient's ultimate discharge destination would be a long-term care setting. The common thread through all these cases is that the value was judged insufficient to justify admission to or continued stay in an acute medical rehabilitation setting.

In addition, as the population has aged, the number of frail elderly persons living in community settings has increased. These individuals often have multiple physical health problems that restrict their functional capacities, but not so severely as to require institutional care. Acute episodes of illness requiring hospitalization exacerbate preexisting functional limitations and prolonged periods of inactivity associated with recovery from illness or surgery result in additional physical debility. Prompt rehabilitative intervention designed to restore functional competence and physical strength and endurance could be the primary determinant of return to the community or need for long-term care. The majority of these "at risk" persons have medical diagnoses that are not included in the diagnostic categories deemed appropriate by the Health Care Financing Administration (HCFA) for admission to medical rehabilitation facilities. For example, persons with chronic cardiac or pulmonary disease that significantly limits their physical capabilities often contract acute illnesses (e.g., pneumonia, influenza) resulting in substantial decline in function and brief hospitalization (e.g., 6 days). At the time of discharge, physical debility frequently has reached the point that return to home is not practical. Alternatively, elderly persons requiring abdominal or gastrointestinal (GI) surgery may be physically incapable of returning home for recovery and convalescence but may be ready for discharge from the hospital. In each of these cases, subacute rehabilitation has become a viable alternative to long-term care placement. Such cases, which can constitute more than half of a subacute rehabilitation case-load, typically are referred to subacute rehabilitation settings for the intensive interdisciplinary services needed to support a return to prior living situations.

Finally, purchasers concerned about the cost of acute medical rehabilitation have sought better value (typically defined by a lower per diem cost) in skilled nursing facilities (SNFs) capable of providing a high level of rehabilitation service. In response, selected SNFs have developed the capacity to provide intensive inpatient rehabilitation to a range of persons with disabilities, including those who conventionally were treated in more expensive acute medical rehabilitation facilities. In these instances, the subacute setting (i.e., the SNF) has become a *venue of care*, providing both acute medical and subacute rehabilitation levels of care.

Rehabilitation is a dynamic learning process. It seeks to promote changes in a person's functional capacities through skill training, therapeutic exercises, and specialized treatments. The mission, culture, and staff expertise in skilled nursing facilities pertain to long-term care rather than rehabilitation. Successful implementation of SNF-based outcome-focused medical rehabilitation requires fundamental paradigm shifts.

PARADIGM SHIFT: SETTING THE VISION

At least two fundamental paradigm shifts are involved in establishing and operating a comprehensive, outcome-focused subacute medical rehabilitation capacity in a SNF. The most obvious is the shift from a long-term care frame of reference to a medical rehabilitative perspective. Less obvious, but no less critical, is the shift from a process-oriented perspective to an outcome-oriented approach.

Shift from Long-Term Care to Rehabilitative Perspective

Excellence in long-term care involves creating an environment that facilitates the maintenance of the highest practicable levels of quality of life for residents. In most cases, the adverse effects of disease or injury have made it impractical for residents of long-term care facilities to meet daily needs associated with living in the community. Long-term care facility staff provide the human support necessary for meeting daily living needs in an institutional setting. High-quality restorative nursing care seeks to minimize or delay the loss of a resident's functional competence by providing opportunities for the long-term care resident to use whatever capacities he or she possesses during the course of a typical week. Temporary declines in function, typically associated with bouts of illness, are overcome through rehabilitative services and follow-up restorative nursing interventions. The outcome of these long-term care services is to enable the resident of the facility to sustain the highest practicable level of functional competence.

In contrast, medical rehabilitation seeks to restore functional competence to persons whose recent illness/injury renders them sufficiently disabled to preclude return to their prior community living setting at this time. The intended outcome is a return to community living. For some persons who previously were extremely frail and restricted in their capacity to meet everyday living needs, a return to community living may be unlikely. Positive outcomes still may be achieved, however, as gains in functional competence associated with a course of aggressive rehabilitation may yield tangible increases in quality of life and reduce burden on caregivers.

The practical differences between a medical rehabilitation perspective and a long-term-care perspective are substantial. The former is characterized by an aggressive, activist approach that seeks to marshal all the person's internal resources to overcome the debilitating effects of illness/injury. The latter requires caring for the needs of the resident who is disabled by the effects of the illness/injury and preventing further decline when possible. The rehabilitation approach teaches the individual to do for one's self, while the long-term care approach seeks to maintain current functional capabilities. The long-term care approach may actually hinder the restoration of lost capacities. Integrating these dramatically different approaches in a single facility is a complex and challenging process.

Before a comprehensive, subacute medical rehabilitation program can be established in a SNF, the administrator, director of nursing, and department heads must first understand the practical consequences in day-to-day operations of adopting a rehabilitation perspective. It is critical that they then clearly communicate to all employees of the long-term care facility the reasons for transforming part of the facility to a subacute medical rehabilitation unit. The subacute unit will require more resources than other parts of the facility, and such resources (e.g., staff, space, systems) typically are scarce or nonexistent in long-term care facilities. Reallocation of already limited resources without clear communication of the reasons can create a perception of a devaluing of the long-term care residents and staff, generate conflict and animosity, and provoke active or passive resistance to the transformation.

One method that has proved useful is to explain the different expectations of the persons served by long-term care facilities and medical rehabilitative facilities. This can be done by leading the institution's management team in the following exercise. The management team is asked to list the facility's benefits as though speaking to a prospective resident and family member. They are then asked to repeat the exercise as though speaking to a family member exploring rehabilitation options for a patient who recently fractured a hip or experienced a stroke. When completing the second part of the exercise the management team usually omits critical features of a rehabilitation facility. For example, long-term care management teams almost never mention the length of stay or discharge rates for persons with similar disabilities, the amount of space available for rehabilitative service delivery, the typical schedule of persons serviced in the subacute rehabilitation unit, or the availability of a nurse liaison to visit the prospective patient at the acute care hospital to review the person's needs and likely treatment plan. This exercise provides the opportunity to discuss the changes that should occur and the practical operational consequences of this shift from long-term care to subacute care. The exercise can be a starting point for actually laying out the operational differences. For example, a long-term care admissions coordinator is primarily a processor of information for people seeking a long-term care bed. A community-based nurse liaison in a subacute setting must communicate information about program benefits and capabilities as they pertain to an individual with specific clinical and social circumstances. The shift from one to the other is challenging (and may not be possible for some people). The recognition of the different demands of staff presented by the subacute patient is a key step toward creating an operational plan to establish and run this new unit.

Each department head can examine the practical implications of the transformation from a long-term care provider to a subacute rehabilitation provider. Establishing a 25-bed subacute rehabilitation unit in a 160-bed SNF likely will result in a tenfold increase in the number of admissions and discharges per month. Marketplace realities also will require that admissions occur in a manner that meets the needs of the referring facility, leading to days with multiple admissions on different shifts. This can be extremely disruptive to personnel in admissions, housekeeping, business office, medical records, and social services, as well as to the nursing and therapy departments. The administrator must prepare the department heads, and they in turn their staffs, for these changes. Clear communication of the overall rationale for reorganizing the facility to compete effectively in the subacute marketplace is critical to easing the burden that will accompany this transformation.

Most long-term care administrators lack the experience required to anticipate all of the operational consequences associated with the business decision to become a subacute provider. In fact, one of the challenges often associated with the conversion to subacute care is that the business decision was made by the owner or operator of the skilled nursing facility. The administrator and the director of nursing may understand the economic incentives for making this business decision but typically be less clear about the substantial challenges that must be overcome to operate a subacute rehabilitation unit successfully. This reality often leads owners and operators of skilled nursing facilities who want to capitalize on the business opportunities associated with subacute care to hire the experts required to operate such units. These experts may be hired as corporate employees, may be consultants, may be management companies, or may be companies that provide all the management and therapy services. Those responsible for opening and operating an SNF-based subacute rehabilitation unit must develop a close working relationship with the facility administrator and director of nursing. In particular, they must provide the necessary technical expertise and guidance, while respecting the administrator's and director of nursing's leadership roles and responsibilities.

On a practical level, an effective working relationship can help overcome the challenges that arise as a result of the differences between long-term care and subacute rehabilitation. When those charged with leading the transformation to subacute care demonstrate the capacity to work through the conflicts, they provide a leadership example to the staff. Establishing and nourishing such a working relationship require mutual respect for each other's expertise. Rehabilitation personnel typically lack a full appreciation of what is required to operate a high-quality long-term care facility in light of tight economic constraints, burdensome regulatory requirements, and personnel challenges. There is a tendency for rehabilitation personnel to act in ways that communicate disregard for and disrespect to seasoned long-term care professionals. This typically is unintentional and arises from ignorance of the realities of long-term care. By focusing on their area of expertise and disregarding the realities of long-term care, rehabilitation personnel unwittingly come across as arrogant, thereby hindering creation of an atmosphere of trust and mutual respect.

Rehabilitation leaders must develop a complete understanding of the pressures and challenges of operating a long-term care facility. These include the Omnibus Budget Reconciliation Act (OBRA) requirements (including resident assessment and care planning using the Minimal Data Set [MDS] and the Resident Assessment Protocols [RAPs]) and the state licensing survey process. Rehabilitation leaders also must understand the fundamental principles of reimbursement and cash flow so they can appreciate the effects of admitting individuals with higher-acuity subacute rehabilitation needs. This is particularly important with respect to the impact of subacute rehabilitation on nursing hours per patient day (NHPPD) for a facility that already has exceeded its routine cost limit. The operating and cost differences between a 2.7 and a 5.5 NHPPD level of care are substantial and represent a significant cash flow issue until the facility is able to get an exception to its routine cost limit to reflect the increased acuity. Rehabilitation leaders with an understanding of the operating realities of a long-term care facility can appreciate the constraints that influence administrators' and nursing directors' decisions and attitudes. This awareness can help rehabilitation leaders adopt a long-term care perspective as they seek to arrive at creative solutions to daily operating challenges in partnership with the administrator and director of nursing.

A rehabilitation leader who is well versed in the realities of operating a long-term care facility also is better prepared to educate therapists about these realities. Creating an interdisciplinary approach to rehabilitation in a skilled nursing facility is an evolutionary process. Therapists recruited from acute medical rehabilitation settings often fail to understand the sources of the cultural and operational differences between long-term care and medical rehabilitation. Frustrations with trying to bridge the cultural and operational gaps may be expressed in ways that alienate long-term care staff. The rehabilitation leader can help foster the environment to translate the subacute vision to reality by educating therapists, demonstrating respect for long-term care personnel, guiding problem solving in the context of a long-term care perspective, counseling patience, celebrating successful evolutionary steps, and supporting therapists when required.

Shift from Process-Oriented Approach to Outcome-Oriented Approach

Long-term care is inherently process-oriented. Unfortunately, rehabilitation historically has tended to be process-oriented as well. Although this process approach has proved successful as indicated by the majority of patients improving sufficiently in functional capacity to support discharge to noninstitutional settings, it has been inefficient. A primary source of this inefficiency is the tendency to treat a wide range of patient impairments and disabilities in a stepwise fashion, building ultimately to an outcome (long-term discharge goal).

Market demands, however, have established new constraints on providers (particularly in the SNF setting), including shorter lengths of stay, reduced reimbursement, and external management of service utilization. These constraints require rehabilitation providers to identify, *at the inception of treatment*, those factors that will affect their capacity to produce valued outcomes. These factors include

- resource availability (e.g., per diem cost allotment, anticipated length of stay, prescribed treatments),
- discharge placement requirements (e.g., site, environmental modifications and human supports, functional competencies),
- current clinical profile and expected recovery curve,
- therapeutic interventions most likely to elicit required functional competencies.

The outcomes-oriented approach to rehabilitation planning and service delivery starts with defining the results that can be expected under a negotiated level and scope of rehabilitation service. Rehabilitation team members must focus their assessments on the degree of change in disability status and functional competence that can be achieved within the given resource constraints. The team must be able to identify and prioritize specific clinical outcomes and selectively apply rehabilitative interventions to overcome barriers to their achievement, including impairments, disabilities, and social factors. The differences between a process-oriented and an outcome-oriented approach are principally a matter of emphasis, focus, and priority. A brief case example may be helpful. A case manager refers a potential admission to the rehabilitation program manager — an 82-year-old woman who had a stroke with resultant left hemiparesis. She was living alone in a ground floor apartment, meals were provided twice daily by Meals on Wheels, and her daughter visited her at least twice a week, assisting her with housework and shopping. The patient had a history of coronary artery disease, with two previous heart attacks. Her walking was limited to residential mobility, and she used a wheelchair for community outings involving more than a short walk. The case manager seeks to determine the realistic probability of the patient's capacity to return to her apartment as she desires. Her daughter voices concern that the added disability associated with the stroke might be the deciding factor in having to consider long-term care placement.

The case manager authorizes a 3-day evaluation period to assess the probabilities of a return to home and the treatment plan that would be required to achieve such an outcome. Therapists following an outcome-oriented approach would focus on

- defining the functional skill requirements to support return to her apartment,
- pinpointing the salient functional skill deficits and impairments that currently preclude her attainment of the functional skill requirements,
- predicting the specific rehabilitation service plan (i.e., type of service, modalities, frequency, intensity, duration of service) that would result in her achieving the functional skill requirements,
- predicting the social and environmental supports required to achieve and sustain a successful return to her apartment,
- predicting the probability of achieving the projected outcome (rehabilitation prognosis).

This approach might rely on many of the same assessment methodologies as a conventional process-oriented approach. However, the assessment team would need to focus, both individually and collectively, on producing the desired information. Similarly, the collective programming of care, if approved by the case manager, would almost exclusively focus on the salient functional skill deficits and impairments identified in the assessment process.

An outcomes-oriented perspective emphasizes disability reduction and identification of treatment priorities that will yield desired outcomes more efficiently. Our experience has taught us not to underestimate the practical challenges associated with reorganizing rehabilitation care planning and service delivery to support an outcomes-oriented approach. In most cases, these practical challenges pertain to people, processes, and systems. We have found that certain themes resonate regardless of the *venue of care* (e.g., inpatient acute rehabilitation, outpatient settings, postacute residential settings, community-based programs, or subacute settings). The *venue of care* typically only affects the way these themes manifest themselves. This section focuses on how we have addressed these challenges in long-term care settings.

People Challenges in Outcome-Oriented Subacute Rehabilitation

Change, even when it is adaptive, causes discomfort in most people. A key feature in helping clinical personnel to manage the distress associated with the shift to an outcome-oriented approach is to emphasize the benefits to the patient of such a change. Most clinicians entered their professions to help people, and many of them perceive that decisions about patient care resulting from market realities are inconsistent with the patient's best interests. In particular, they resent what they perceive as a minimalist approach, in which care is tightly restricted to limited areas of daily functioning, with outcome goals limited to discharge to a less expensive level of care, regardless of a patient's potential or need. This is in stark contrast to the approach in which patients receive a broad range of rehabilitative services designed to yield the greatest benefit to the patient and family for as long as tangible evidence of progress is apparent.

Long-term care settings with subacute rehabilitation capacity are increasingly being selected as lower cost alternatives to acute medical rehabilitation settings by managed care entities. Per diem reimbursement rates typically are quite modest compared to acute medical rehabilitation rates. Aggressive utilization review practices result in very short lengths of stay, restrictions on which disciplines are authorized to treat a patient, and, in many cases, limits on daily service intensity. These practices often reflect the minimalist approach, giving rise to substantial operating challenges for the therapists.

For example, we tell our therapists that the outcome-oriented approach to rehabilitation care planning and service delivery is the method most likely to deliver value to the patient and family. We begin by orienting our therapists to our clinical philosophy, which establishes TheraTx as a rehabilitation provider committed to producing the best value. We instruct our therapists to "provide no more than, but no less than, the level of rehabilitation service required to achieve the *best outcome* for the patient/family *within available resources.*" Our clinical philosophy is aligned with the value system of our clinicians, yet is tempered by the economic realities established by the purchaser. It provides the vehicle for stimulating discussion of how to achieve the highest level of effectiveness and efficiency, regardless of resource constraints. Discussion of our philosophy leads to an explanation of how we have incorporated the outcome-oriented approach into our service delivery model. In this context, we find greater willingness to accept the discomfort associated with learning a new approach.

For the professional and paraprofessional SNF staff accustomed to serving the needs of long-term care residents, the changes associated with the addition of a subacute rehabilitation program are substantial. The apparently minor distinction between the terms *resident* and *patient* denotes the different focus of the long-term care and subacute units. All too often these terms have dramatically different connotations, with *patient* implying a "higher status" in the minds of rehabilitation personnel. The patient is transitioning to the community, and his or her rehabilitation is more important than the long-term resident's, since he or she is already in an institutional setting designed to care for his or her needs.

An outcomes-oriented approach emphasizes functional recovery, regardless of the patient's projected living arrangement following a course of rehabilitation. Outcome (i.e., improved functional competence; reduced burden on caregivers) is just as important to a long-term care resident as it is to a subacute rehabilitation patient. Advocating an outcomes-oriented approach for all persons in the skilled nursing facility, whether short-term patients or long-term residents, helps overcome the emotional resistance to change associated with incorporating subacute programs in a skilled nursing facility.

One of the greatest sources of distress experienced by long-term care personnel is the change in the pace of doing one's job. Virtually every aspect of daily operations is strained by the introduction of subacute rehabilitation patients. The volume of admissions and discharges increases dramatically, and the response times needed to satisfy market expectations are substantially shorter than when dealing with long-term care admissions. The acuity of the patients' conditions requires greater nursing resources, both in NHPPD and in clinical expertise. Social services must work closely and rapidly with families to ensure that details relevant to discharge are managed effectively. Nursing aides must ensure that subacute patients are ready for scheduled therapy sessions. This includes refraining from "doing for" the patient so that therapy occurs as part of naturally occurring events such as getting up, grooming, dressing, and eating. To make matters worse, nursing staff typically earn no more for serving subacute patients, despite the added performance requirements.

The stress associated with the change to subacute care for the long-term care personnel can be managed, in part, through clarification of outcome expectations, resource constraints, and essential conditions affecting discharge within defined time parameters. As a practical matter, this understanding must be translated into a daily operational plan to address any and all critical factors that affect achievement of the expected outcome. We employ a daily "stand-up" meeting in which key team members review critical patient management and care coordination issues. The meeting typically takes place adjacent to the nursing station with all participants standing. This discourages long meetings while ensuring that critical concerns are communicated and acted upon by designated point persons. Keeping patient outcomes in the forefront of these discussions helps foster interdisciplinary cooperation at the most pragmatic level—"Who is going to take care of this critical issue today?" It also helps long-term care personnel focus on what needs to be done to improve operating efficiencies and to address "system failures" instead of attributing breakdowns in coordination of care to "people failures."

Another major source of stress associated with an outcomes-oriented approach is that therapists and nurses accustomed to working in long-term care settings typically are not used to integrating assessment findings to project likely recovery rates under specific resource constraints and restricted levels of service provision. There is little impetus to develop and apply such skills to the management of the long-term resident's needs, since predicting the rate of recovery or the degree of functional change associated with a given amount and type of rehabilitative intervention are not viewed as relevant issues when servicing long-term care residents. Even though therapists recruited to subacute rehabilitation units in SNFs from rehabilitation facilities are more accustomed to projecting level of functioning at discharge, when pressed by third party payer representatives to defend their rationale for requested increases in service utilization, they become less secure about linking the expected incremental gains in functional competence and their impact on ongoing burden of care to the additional resource expenditure. Finally, given the shortages of skilled therapists, it is not uncommon that relatively inexperienced therapists (e.g., less than 2 years experience) are asked to make projections that neither their clinical training nor their practice experience prepared them to make.

An outcomes-oriented approach can provide a remedy to the dilemmas noted. We have found that the change to such an approach provides the framework for thinking about the critical data that should be collected in an assessment so that projections about outcome expectations in various service utilization scenarios can be made with reasonable levels of validity. In essence, an outcome-oriented approach results in an outcome-focused assessment as contrasted to a clinical profile of impairment and disability scores. We also have discovered that seasoned therapists respond to the challenge to interpret the meaning of their findings, rather than merely reporting them and proceeding with standard approaches to care for distinct diagnostic groups. The outcome-oriented approach provides a framework for converting clinical findings into tailored treatment plans. Moreover, these more experienced therapists can be paired with more inexperienced therapists as mentors. Finally, we have created a clinical database that facilitates feedback to clinicians about the relationships between service utilization and functional change for a variety of clinical populations.

Process Challenges in Outcome-Oriented Subacute Rehabilitation

One of the most vexing integration challenges faced by management and staff in SNFs that develop subacute rehabilitation programs involves the federally mandated resident assessment instrument (RAI). The RAI has three components: the Minimum Data Set (MDS), the Resident Assessment Protocols (RAPs), and the utilization guidelines specified in the State Operations Manual (SOM) 241. The RAI was developed in response to the OBRA 1987 mandate to develop and implement a uniform system to assess a long-term care resident's ability to perform daily living functions and to identify significant impairments. The MDS and RAPs data are the basis for developing and implementing plans of care to ensure that each resident achieves and sustains the highest practicable levels of physical, mental, and psychosocial functioning.

The MDS is a uniform screening tool designed to discern whether any of 18 specified conditions or combinations of conditions should be addressed via a care-plan intervention. The RAPs form a structured assessment process designed to identify the nature and causes of the 18 conditions "triggered" by the MDS. This is a problem-oriented approach to functional assessment that provides the structure through the RAP guidelines to determine what, if any, clinical management or treatment interventions should be instituted.

This process is required to be completed upon admission to a SNF, and then at least annually and at any "significant change" in resident status unrelated to transitory events. A quarterly review of resident status must be conducted to ensure that the MDS findings are still reflective of resident status.

The initial MDS is based upon a common baseline observation period, typically 7 days prior to a specified assessment date. This date can be no later than the 14th day following admission, but is typically earlier since the RAP process must also be completed no later than day 14. An initial plan of care should be developed within 48 hours of admission, but the formal plan of care based on the MDS and RAPs must be completed within 21 days of admission.

Persons admitted to SNFs for short-term subacute rehabilitation expect to be discharged to community settings after a relatively short stay. Rehabilitation lengths of stay (RLOS) typically average less than 45 days for most disability groups. For example, a recent review of nearly 10,000 subacute rehabilitation patients serviced by TheraTx revealed an average RLOS of 25 days for a population predominantly recovering from stroke, orthopedic, and a range of general medical conditions.

The MDS and RAPs processes were not designed to guide the assessment and care planning process for such patients. Conventional rehabilitation practice and marketplace expectations dictate that formal rehabilitation assessments be completed within 48 hours of admission, with interim care plans reviewed and revised within 7 days. There is a reasonable expectation of significant progress in response to rehabilitation service delivery each week. Absence of significant changes in functional status over a 21-day period would typically be cause to discontinue aggressive rehabilitation.

Conventional approaches to functional assessment utilized by rehabilitation professionals and third party payers to determine medical necessity and whether the reasonable expectation of progress standard is being satisfied (e.g., Functional Independence Measure [FIM], Level of Rehabilitation Scale [LORS], Patient Evaluation Conference System [PECS]) are not employed in the pertinent MDS sections. The MDS is a screening tool designed to identify conditions that might indicate the need for skilled rehabilitation services based on global measures of cognition, communication, physical functioning, nutritional status, and skin condition. The findings reflect typical levels of performance across a 7-day observation period. Given the purpose for which it was designed and its measurement methods, it is, not surprisingly, inadequate for the purpose of assessing functional skill levels of short-term rehabilitation patients and the nature and extent of progress in response to brief, intensive skilled therapy.

The incompatibility of the assessment and care planning process with the needs of the long-term care and subacute populations often leads to parallel processes. For example, nursing, social service, dietary, and activities personnel complete the MDS and RAPs to satisfy federal mandates to prevent deficiencies during the state survey process. This activity may or may not lead to a formal care plan since many of the subacute rehabilitation patients are already discharged within 21 days of admission, and even if a care plan is developed, it often has little or no bearing on rehabilitation service delivery. The rehabilitation team members serving the subacute unit simply conduct parallel rehabilitation meetings to define the nature and amount of rehabilitative care to be delivered to the patient.

A more satisfying solution is to develop a single, outcomes-oriented approach to assessment and care planning for subacute rehabilitation patients. Within 24 hours of admission each discipline conducts a formal assessment, which is documented in the patient's chart. Prior to the initial team conference (no later than 7 days after admission), the MDS is completed by nursing, dietary, activities, and social service personnel. Therapy documentation (initial assessments and progress notes) provides the basis for the RAPs for all pertinent triggered conditions (e.g., ADL functional/rehabilitation potential, cognitive loss/dementia, communication, nutritional status). Critical patient management issues are communicated among team members in the daily stand-up meeting. Thus, by the time the team convenes in a formal patient care plan meeting, they have all the necessary information to confirm outcome expectations. The primary interdisciplinary communication should be centered on consensus regarding the patient's likely disability status at discharge, likely ongoing human and environmental support requirements, and timing of discharge.

Another key topic of interdisciplinary communication should focus on what all team members must do to reinforce patient learning. The generalization of skill learning beyond the formal therapy session is critical, especially in circumstances of constrained resources. Ensuring that all staff consistently use the same technique and in all situations in which the patient must perform a behavior has always been a challenge in rehabilitation settings. This is compounded in SNFs, where the result of staffing ratios and conventional practice is that nursing aides perform tasks for the person instead of supporting the person in learning self-competence. We have found that programming for generalization in SNF environments requires ongoing practical inservicing of nursing personnel; focus on a few very critical behaviors and techniques; simple, direct communication of the way to support the person's learning; and routine rounds to ensure that such procedures are occurring. Needless to say, this entire effort is fruitless without the full support of nursing administration. We have found that emphasizing the need to maximize patient learning to achieve outcome goals in increasingly shorter time frames is the best way to elicit such support.

The critical components of this approach for subacute rehabilitation patients are displayed in Figure 6–1. The processes and time frames evolve over time. In our experience, each facility wants to use its own formats for communication among team members, for charting, and for care plans. Managing patient care effectively and efficiently is the success strategy, as contrasted to worrying about what form or format is used.

The process as outlined for subacute rehabilitation patients differs from the process used for long-term care residents. Principal differences include the following:

- The initial MDS observation period typically does not begin until day 3 or 4.
- Outcome expectations do not include relatively rapid return to community living, reducing both the range of issues that must be managed and the need for rapid collection and assimilation of information and formulation of action plans to facilitate discharge.
- Once immediate resident management issues and methods are clarified, there is no practical need for daily stand-up meeting reviews.

Nurse liaison conducts *on site clinical review.* Outcome expectations outlined including patient/family and payer parameters.

Pre-Admission

Disciplines initiate *clinical assessments.* Identify immediate patient management issues & methods. *MDS observation* period begins.

Admission Day

Initial *"stand-up" meeting:*
- Critical patient management /social issues communicated to all team members.
- Initial read on probability of achieving patient/family & payer outcome expectations.
- Red flag any major barriers to outcome attainment and develop plan to address issue(s).

Complete assessments; initiate provisional care plan.

Day 2

Proceed with implementation of *provisional care plan* and *MDS observation* at discipline level.

Stand-up meeting:
- Note any patient management issues
- Communicate specific suggestions from team members re: patient management methods
- Debrief team on findings re: "red flag" outcome issue(s).

Day 3

Stand-up meeting:
- Identify any issue requiring modification of provisional care plans based on patient management or social issues. Otherwise proceed as outlined in discipline-specific goals.
- Discuss need for home evaluation & potential schedule.

Rounds: Initial review with nursing aide & charge nurse of patient performance during walking rounds on unit. Discuss any inconsistencies/ concerns raised in MDS observation.

Day 4

Complete MDS & RAPs: Identify critical problems, goals, interventions online with provisional care plans.

Initial team conference to:
- validate/modify patient care plan based on first week of response to treatment and observation of performance capacities.
- modify individual discipline's interim plans and focus as warranted.
- communicate "success" interventions, especially methods to be used by other team members; seek advice re: difficult patient management issues.
- target selected "critical" behaviors for entire staff to focus upon and specific intervention plan for aide level staff.
- develop definitive discharge plan and action steps to address any issues pertaining to discharge.
- establish probable discharge date.

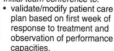

Day 5–7

Daily stand-up meeting:
- Note any changes in patient plan dictated by clinical condition, response to treatment, social circumstances or payer requirements.
- Identify action steps required to ensure outcome attainment other than clinical improvement of patient in response to treatment.

Weekly walking rounds:
Ensure that selected "critical" behaviors are actually being addressed on unit according to defined methods.

Weekly patient care conference:
- Confirm rate of progress within expected parameters
- Identify concerns relative to achieving projected level of functional competence/health
- Alter intervention plans as warranted
- Confirm action steps completed and assign new action steps re: any concerns about achieving planned discharge. Modify discharge plan and date if necessary
- Order equipment & schedule postdischarge services

Family/caregiver training
Initiate as early as feasible. Timing based on family's "need to know" to facilitate outcome as anticipated.

Day 8–ff

Figure 6–1 An Outcome-Oriented Approach to Subacute Rehabilitation Programming

- Review of resident performance in rounds is far less frequent and less aggressive since the expectation for substantive change in a relatively brief time frame is not present.
- The initial care plan meeting may not be formalized until the third week of a long-term care resident's stay.
- The primary focus of care planning and intervention is sustaining the resident's functional competence or forestalling decline rather than eliciting substantial improvement in functional capacities as with subacute rehabilitation patients.
- The initial observation period is longer and focuses on the resident's life style preferences and ways of adapting to his or her new living environment.

The suggested revisions in the assessment and care planning process for subacute rehabilitation patients are completely consistent with the intent of OBRA to ensure that these patients achieve their highest practicable level of functioning during the course of their SNF stay. The mandated MDS is completed, the RAPs process occurs and is documented, and care plans focus on what is necessary to ensure maximal functional skill improvements. Time frames for collecting MDS data, ways of documenting the RAPs process, and formats of care plans may be different for subacute rehabilitation and long-term care residents, but the promotion of the highest quality of care through a coordinated, interdisciplinary team approach is consistent throughout the facility.

System Challenges in Outcome-Oriented Subacute Rehabilitation

Systems are integral tools for operating an outcome-driven service, and information management is a key component of personnel and program management. We have developed an integrated automated information management system (TheraSys) to meet these needs. A detailed description of this system is beyond the scope of this chapter. We will instead focus on system components and uses that enable us to manage our subacute rehabilitation programs to produce value.

Our experience with guiding clinicians to an outcomes-oriented perspective has taught us that changing patient documentation systems to reflect such a perspective is exceptionally important. We emphasize disability reduction, since a person's functional competence is a fundamental determinant of the capacity to manage daily living needs and the burden associated with ongoing support requirements. The value of rehabilitation is heavily influenced by the extent to which services rendered produced change in the person's disability status.

We have arranged our patient documentation system to focus each clinician on functional behaviors in a number of ways. First, we require our therapists to rate patient performance in a range of behaviors essential for everyday living, such as fall recovery, residential mobility, and community mobility, in addition to more conventional mobility items. We focus on specific communicative behaviors instead of rating expressive and receptive language. We arrange the layout of our documentation to highlight disability scores, rather than impairment ratings such as range of motion, strength, muscle tone, balance, endurance, or length of utterances.

Clinicians tend to focus on impairments, in both assessment and treatment. Moreover, the connection between an individual's impairments and his or her disability status is rarely made explicit by therapists. Our approach to outcomes-oriented rehabilitation led us to create a means for therapists to indicate the practical significance of a patient's impairments. This method involves each therapist's selecting the patient's principal underlying impairments (e.g., musculoskeletal, sensory, perceptual, cognitive, communicative, psychological) from a standard glossary of impairments. The therapist then describes the practical significance of an impairment such as limited range of motion on each of the disability items (e.g., eating, dressing, grooming). This is done by using an impairment impact scale. The end result of this process is a clinical matrix that summarizes the patient's clinical profile, with a primary focus on disability and impairment impact. In other words, the structure of the documentation system supports an outcomes-oriented perspective.

The clinical matrix is completed at admission and weekly until discharge. These data form part of a relational database that also includes all relevant information on rehabilitative service utilization and costs, detailed to the level of an individual patient and therapist. Patient demographic and diagnostic information also is a component of this database. Standardized management reports are produced by the system on a real-time basis, permitting program staff to manage all aspects of service delivery to yield targeted clinical and fiscal outcomes. We believe that such information management tools are essential to operate an outcome-oriented rehabilitation program, whether in an SNF, a hospital, a rehabilitation facility, or a community-based program. Such systems are especially important in an SNF, since the long-term care industry as a rule has been slow to adopt integrated, automated management information systems.

It is crucial to make a substantial investment in information technology for a variety of reasons, including enhancing the care provided by our clinicians. There is substantial variability in skill and experience among therapists, especially in the area of predicting the relationship between a given amount and type of therapeutic intervention and disability reduction. This is true for given populations (e.g., elective hip replacement and fractured hip patient groups), as well as individual patients. By collecting a wide range of clinical, demographic, diagnostic, service utilization, and cost data in a relational database, we can help individual clinicians to identify likely outcomes for a given type of patient assuming a certain type and amount of rehabilitative intervention. For example, consider three hemiplegic stroke patients, each of whom requires maximal assistance in most functional mobility and ADL behaviors. All had unremarkable prestroke histories. Assume that in the first case the assessment data revealed that the primary underlying impairments were paresis, weakness, limited range of motion, and impaired sitting and standing balance. In the second case, assume that the assessment data revealed that the primary underlying impairments were paresis, impaired proprioceptive and kinesthetic feedback, hemispatial neglect, impaired motor learning, and impaired safety awareness. Finally, assume that the third patient presented the same pattern of impairments as the second patient, but with greater severity. Our system requires our therapists to rate the degree to which the underlying impairments impact negatively on the functional behaviors (e.g., grooming). In this example, assume that the impairment impact rating revealed that the average impairment impact ratings for patient two ranged from the minor to the moderate impact level, whereas the third patient's impairment impact ratings were in the severe to extreme level. These three left hemiplegic stroke patients with relatively equivalent disability levels upon admission will require significantly different levels and types of rehabilitation interventions, resulting in very different resource utilization patterns. In addition, their lengths of stay, levels of functional competence at discharge, and probability of return to prior living circumstances likely will be quite different. Our goal is to aggregate sufficient data on a broad range of subacute rehabilitation patients to provide guidelines to therapists regarding predicted outcomes (clinical and financial) given patient profile at admission. The use of information systems goes beyond prediction. An even more critical function is the identification of "best clinical practices" and the redesign of the way we provide therapy. We refer to this process as clinical process engineering.

Clinical Process Engineering

Clinical process engineering involves the following steps:
- Define targeted clinical outcome(s).
- Determine the service components essential to produce the desired results.
- Develop programs and protocols incorporating essential service components.
- Train clinical staff to focus on targeted outcomes and to execute clinical programs effectively to achieve outcomes.
- Use information technology to monitor activities, costs, and outcomes and use information to improve clinical processes.
- Redesign clinical activities to reduce work requirements and minimize labor costs.

For example, the outputs from the clinical database reveal that a particular facility achieved better-than-average performance with hip replacement patients, in terms of functional mobility change scores, levels of functional independence at discharge, and length of stay and rehabilitation charges. Consultation with the program personnel revealed that they had modified the standard protocols of care in the following ways:
- Physical therapists focused on the design of technical interventions required to support functional mobility changes and supervision of physical therapy (PT) assistants and rehabilitation technicians.
- Physical therapists spent concentrated time educating patients about how nursing aides and rehabilitation technicians should be assisting them. Patients were instructed not to permit an aide to do a task that they could do with proper assistance.
- The rehabilitation technician conducted daily rounds across two shifts reviewing specific assistance methods and promoting opportunities for the patient to perform daily living tasks (e.g., bed mobility, transfers, walking).

- Early in the stay (typically by day 3) physical therapists reviewed with family members critical factors in ongoing support requirements, specific assistance methods, and family encouragement of the patient's performing everyday living tasks as much as possible.

In summary, rehabilitation team members had reengineered the way care was provided. The initial impetus for this change were utilization constraints placed on therapy by managed care representatives. The positive outcomes caused the approach to be expanded to all patients, regardless of resource availability. The lessons learned at this "best practice" facility would then be disseminated to all other facilities. Subsequent monitoring of performance in all buildings would reveal the extent to which the best practice had been replicated successfully in other sites.

We believe that clinical process engineering will lead to continual improvements in program effectiveness and efficiency. Simply automating clinical and financial systems is insufficient to produce the operating efficiencies we anticipate will be required when servicing managed care patients. We believe that a fundamental reorganization of the planning and delivery of care, guided by the clinical process engineering approach, is necessary.

CONCLUSION

We have attempted to address pragmatic issues associated with creating and operating a subacute rehabilitation program in SNF settings. An outcome-oriented approach has provided the framework for addressing the operational challenges experienced across a rapidly growing network of approximately 120 sites. It is an evolutionary process and we hope that others who are currently engaged in this process will benefit from reflecting on our experience.

Chapter 7

Preparing Rehabilitation Teams for Outcome-Based Rehabilitation

Nancy D. Schmidt, MS

Objectives

- To provide rehabilitation managers with tools for preparing staff to shift into an outcome-based service delivery model.
- To address the role of senior management in supporting interdisciplinary outcome-based rehabilitation.
- To present strategies for organizing and training staff for outcome-based rehabilitation.

INTRODUCTION

Providing outcome-based rehabilitation requires a shift in the way rehabilitation is conceptualized, organized, and delivered. It requires clinicians to become "managers of outcome" in addition to being "care-givers." Outcome-based rehabilitation requires a change in thinking about the priorities and focus of rehabilitation. This shift may be challenging for rehabilitation managers, supervisors, and clinicians who were trained in the traditional service-based rehabilitation model. My purpose in this chapter is to provide information to rehabilitation leaders and managers about how to prepare staff to shift into an outcome-based service delivery model. The following areas will be reviewed:

- The importance of leading and managing the organization from an outcome-based perspective
- Senior management's role in supporting interdisciplinary teams toward outcome-based rehabilitation
- Organizing and training of staff for outcome-based rehabilitation
- Staff instruction on how to work with families from an outcome-based perspective

LEADING THE ORGANIZATION FROM AN OUTCOMES PERSPECTIVE

Leaders who decide to move outcome-based rehabilitation must begin by modeling an outcome approach in their management of the organization. Leading the organization from an outcome approach is thoroughly reviewed in O'Lear's chapter and therefore will not be detailed within the scope of this chapter.

It is important for staff to have leaders and managers who are clear and honest in their description of the anticipated outcome of the rehabilitation organization. Questions that must be addressed include

1. What is the purpose of the rehabilitation organization?
2. What is the mission? Is it different from the purpose?
3. How will the success of the rehabilitation organization be measured?
4. Whom does the rehabilitation organization serve?
5. What are the goals and objectives, quarterly, annually, in 5 years?

The organization's strategic plan that guides its outcome must also be shared with staff. The important factor in communicating this information to staff is the modeling of "front end decision making" (O'Lear, Chapter 8), a concept that is necessary in providing outcome-based rehabilitation.

Other principles involved in outcome management are measuring performance, assessing the environment, assessing customer needs, articulating values, developing an operations plan, and implementing routine audits of the system. When the organization's leaders and managers demonstrate these principles through behavior and action plans, they send a powerful message to staff about the value placed on outcome-oriented planning and decision making.

Managing the outcome of rehabilitation and managing the outcome of an organization involve very similar principles. For example, when leaders embark upon a business plan and fail to inform staff about the purpose, value, mission, and implications of the plan for the organization and staff, staff may react with suspicion and anger. Similarly, when rehabilitation teams embark on a discharge plan for their client and fail to gain family input or fail to provide adequate information about the goals and intended result of the discharge plan, families may react to the team with suspicion and anger.

Often, clinicians and administrators view each other's work as completely foreign. Behind closed doors, clinicians and administrators may comment about one another, "They just don't have a clue" or "If they only had to work a day in my world." Successful outcome-based rehabilitation organizations manage the business of rehabilitation from an outcome perspective. They articulate the value, goal, and outcome of the organization on the basis of its purpose and mission. The organization's action plan and long-range and short-term goals support the projected outcome. The practice of managing the business of rehabilitation for results models the principle of managing rehabilitation outcomes to the rehabilitation team. The two are not mutually exclusive.

SENIOR MANAGEMENT'S ROLE IN SUPPORTING INTERDISCIPLINARY TEAMS TOWARD OUTCOME-BASED REHABILITATION

Senior management must play a vital role in creating an environment that facilitates outcome-based rehabilitation. In fact, without the support and "buying in" of senior management, the rehabilitation organization cannot shift into outcome-based rehabilitation. Specific areas in which senior management staff must commit themselves in order to facilitate an outcome approach to rehabilitation include the following:

- Communicating to staff the value and purpose of moving into outcome-based rehabilitation and the intended results for the organization (Haffey, Chapter 6).
- Committing to provide cost-efficient rehabilitation outcomes. Cost-efficient outcomes entail providing the services necessary to achieve the outcome within the agreed-upon time frame. Providing more or less service and extending lengths of stay without clear rationale or

because the census is low violate this commitment. The rehabilitation team needs to know that a commitment to cost-efficient outcomes is taken seriously and does not change according to the needs or whims of the organization. Admission and discharge criteria should reflect a commitment to cost-efficient outcome.

- Gaining alignment and commitment among physicians to lead outcome-based rehabilitation in organizations in which physicians lead the team and provide focus for the rehabilitation plan. Physicians must be educated and trained on how to lead the team in providing a functional outcome instead of focusing on rehabilitating the patient's impairment. If physicians do not lead from an outcome perspective, the rehabilitation team will be unable to proceed to outcome-based rehabilitation service delivery.

- Ensuring that case managers are seen as leaders of outcome-based rehabilitation. Within many rehabilitation organizations, case management serves as the central organizing force for coordinating services and communication. Because the role of case management is vital in keeping all consumers informed of the rehabilitation plan and progress, case managers must also be trained in the outcome-based model and in leading the team to outcome-based decision making.

- Allocating sufficient time to initial inservices and ongoing follow-up training. Shifting to outcome-based rehabilitation requires a commitment to train management, supervisory personnel, and clinical staff. Training may include bringing in outside expertise or utilizing internal staff.

- Making a financial commitment to allocating necessary resources involved in developing and implementing a system of outcome data collection. Outcome-oriented rehabilitation requires a commitment to a longitudinal outcome tracking system. An outcome tracking system becomes the performance measure in addition to a program evaluation tool. Both are necessary tools, but are costly to set up and maintain.

ORGANIZING AND TRAINING STAFF TO AN OUTCOME ORIENTATION

In order to make the shift into outcome-based rehabilitation, staff will need to have an understanding of the value of making this shift. A good way to begin is to involve them in inservice training that focuses on six issues that form the basis for outcome-based rehabilitation.

1. What is an outcome, and how is it different from a discharge plan?
2. What is a successful outcome? How is success measured?
3. What are the rehabilitation methods used to produce an outcome? When is remediation used versus compensation?
4. What is the difference between patient-centered versus discipline-centered care?
5. How do we form an "alignment" of expectation among the patient, the family, the team, and the payer regarding outcome?
6. What are the differences among impairment, disability, and handicap?

Leading staff toward consensus congruent with the outcome model of rehabilitation within these areas is an important first step in preparing them for understanding outcome-based rehabilitation.

Understanding the Concept

The first step in training an interdisciplinary team about outcome-based rehabilitation is to explain the shift from service-based rehabilitation to outcome-based rehabilitation. Most rehabilitation clinicians' training was influenced by the medical model. This model adheres to the following procedures as related to diagnosis and treatment planning.

Assess/Diagnose ⇨ Treat ⇨ Wait for Result ⇨ Discharge

In outcome-based rehabilitation, the sequence is altered to

Assess/Identify Skill Requirement for Success in the Discharge Setting ⇨ Project Outcome ⇨ Define Barriers ⇨ Define Resources Available ⇨ Manage for Results

This shift must happen in the context of thorough information about the discharge environment. The assessment stage includes assessment of the discharge setting. If the client is returning home, this task is made easier than when discharge to home is not an option. In the latter case, the discharge environment must be identified as soon as possible.

In service-based rehabilitation, the rehabilitation team prioritizes resources around remediating deficits or impairments resulting from an injury. In outcome-based rehabilitation the focus is on reducing "handicapping conditions" that challenge clients' abilities to resume their premorbid life role.

Case Comparison

A useful training activity to help staff differentiate between traditional medical rehabilitation and an outcome-based model is walking them through a case comparison such as the following.

Marie is a 52-year-old married woman who is 3 weeks post onset of a traumatic brain injury sustained from a motor vehicle accident in which she was the driver. Her initial computed tomographic (CT) scan revealed the presence of a right frontal lobe hematoma. She had a Glasgow Coma Scale score of 5 on admission to the emergency room. She was transferred from the intensive care unit (ICU) to the neurotrauma unit on day 5. She became medically stabilized and progressed from a Rancho Level II/III to a Rancho Level IV. She was transferred to an acute rehabilitation facility by day 22.

Marie's husband is in good health and plans to care for her when she returns home with the help of in-home services. Their children are grown and reside in another state. Marie and her husband live in a two-story home with the bedrooms on the second floor. There are a half bath on the first floor and a full bath on the second floor. Marie's husband is semiretired and works 20 hours a week outside the home. This income is necessary for their livelihood. Marie was a homemaker and socially active in her community.

Marie exhibits balance and coordination problems and upper extremity weakness on the left side. She shows significant deficits in attention, short- and long-term memory, and general cognitive decline affecting her judgment and decision-making abilities. She is evaluated as having visual perceptual difficulties that impact her ambulation as well as her writing. She can feed and dress herself with cues, although she cannot be left alone safely for more than 5 minutes because she will attempt to walk alone and may fall. She is disoriented topographically but recognizes family members. She is unable to prepare simple meals as a result of cognitive and perceptual problems. Her language skills are mildly impaired and she is medically stable. Marie is inconsistently continent of bowel and bladder. She becomes mildly agitated upon awakening and again in the early evening. She responds well to redirection. She is estimated to be functioning at Rancho Level IV/V.

Service-Based Rehabilitation Plan

- *Environment in which rehabilitation will occur:* inpatient acute rehabilitation center with follow-up outpatient therapies
- *Rehabilitation goal:* independence in the home environment and in her community
- *Rehabilitation plan:*
  - Physical therapy (PT): 2 times a day for 1 hour to work on balance, coordination, and ambulation
  - Occupational therapy (OT): 2 times per day for activities of daily living (ADL) training and visual perceptual remediation
  - Speech: 2 times per day to remediate attention and memory deficits; remediation of judgment and problem-solving skills
  - Psychiatry/psychology: 3 to 5 times per week for adjustment issues and medication management around behavioral problems if necessary.
  - Nursing: development of a program to increase continence
  - Neuropsychological evaluation: identification of cognitive and behavioral deficits
  - Social service: meeting with the family before discharge to answer questions and to prepare family for the discharge transition; home visit about 1 week before discharge
  - Vocational rehabilitation: not required
- *Estimated length of stay:* 8–10 weeks inpatient, with follow-up services as outpatient for 3 months
- *Inpatient cost:* $850 per day/at 10 weeks = $59,500
- *Outpatient cost:* $650 per day/at 3 times/week for 16 weeks = $31,200
- *Total cost:* $90,700

Outcome-Based Rehabilitation Plan

Projected Outcome Based on Evaluation

Functional independence in self-care, mobility, safety, communication, and home and community integration is the projected outcome. Marie will require the use of a checklist in order to initiate and sequence self-care activities. She will require assistance one time a week to help her plan and structure community activities, such as grocery shopping, trips to the YWCA, and social activities. This structure and planning will be provided by her husband.

The plan will take several factors into account.

- *Environment in which rehabilitation will occur:* inpatient acute rehabilitation followed by home-based rehabilitation
- *Estimated length of stay:* 3 weeks inpatient, 3 weeks home rehabilitation services, and follow-up outpatient appointments
- *Inpatient cost:* $850 per day/at 3 weeks = $17,850
- *Home-based cost:* $450 per day/4 times per week for 2 weeks 3 times per week for 2 weeks = $6,300
- *Outpatient cost:* for family/patient support group for psychosocial adjustment, weekly for 6 weeks = $660
- *Total cost* = $24,810

Inpatient Rehabilitation Goal

Immediate goals of rehabilitation are specified.

1. Marie will acquire safety skills sufficient to support leaving her alone in her home environment alone for up to 30 minutes.
2. Marie will be able to climb a flight of eight stairs with someone standing by to assist in case she needs help.
3. Marie will be able to demonstrate that she can access help in an emergency.
4. Marie will be consistently continent of bowel and bladder.
5. Marie will be able to feed and dress herself independently utilizing a checklist to help her initiate and sequence steps.

Rehabilitation Plan

The patient will be involved in the AM Care (routine morning care) group to work on ADLs and self-feeding. This activity will occur daily. This group is led by OT and nursing. The goal is that Marie will be able to get up, shower, and dress herself with the assistance of intermittent verbal cues to keep her directed.

The patient will work on ambulation in the following ways:

1. She will participate six times a week in the functional mobility group co-led by physical therapy and a certified occupational therapy assistant.

2. She will have individual sessions of physical therapy, 30 minutes per day, 6 days per week, to work on stair climbing. The goal is to climb eight stairs by herself. She will need someone to stand by for safety and balance control for the first 4 weeks.

3. Marie will access help in the event of an emergency. The speech pathologist will work with her toward setting up a consistent set of procedures that she will be taught to follow.

4. Neuropsychology will provide all therapists with a protocol on sustaining attention to functional task.

5. Psychiatry will assess whether Marie is a candidate for pharmacological intervention for the management of her attention disorder. Psychosocial adjustment issues will be identified by psychiatry staff and will begin to be addressed through the family/patient support group.

6. A home visit will be completed in week 1 with Marie and her physical and occupational therapists to evaluate safety in Marie's natural home environment by the middle of week 2. Marie's husband will be involved in teaching by the beginning of week 2 from all therapy staff. A day pass with a performance checklist of areas for home safety will be given to Marie's husband for performance monitoring, which will be initiated on the weekend of week 2.

7. By the beginning of week 3 all therapists will focus on modifying treatment protocols to address problems that may have surfaced during the day pass.

8. During week 3 the home-based therapist will cotreat with the inpatient therapist, review protocols for home-based treatment techniques, and meet with Marie and her husband. The home-based program will be outlined.

9. Marie will be discharged to home on Friday of week 3. Case Management will communicate with Marie's husband daily to obtain progress updates and to begin arranging for in-home services by the end of week 1.

Case Summary

The case compares traditional medical rehabilitation to an outcome-based model. The primary differences in the two approaches may be viewed as follows:

SERVICE-BASED REHABILITATION

- Assesses the patient's impairments
- Defines assessment parameters according to the discipline

- Organizes the treatment plan around patient limitations

OUTCOME-BASED REHABILITATION

- Utilizes a patient-centered assessment
- Defines assessment parameters by the discharge environment; focuses on skill requirements of discharge environment
- Organizes treatment plan around skill requirements of the discharge setting

SERVICE-BASED REHABILITATION

- Focuses treatment on reduction of impairments that underlie skill; remediates first and compensates as last resort
- Sets discipline-based goals

- Provides family teaching at the time of discharge

- Assumes skill generalization

OUTCOME-BASED REHABILITATION

- Focuses treatment on functional skill reacquisition; considers compensation first
- Sets functional goals based on the outcome result to be achieved
- Begins family teaching at admission and continues throughout duration of the treatment (First item taught to family is what an outcome is)
- Builds skill generalization into the treatment plan

ESSENTIAL TOOLS FOR PROVIDING OUTCOME-BASED REHABILITATION

Once staff have an understanding of the conceptual shift inherent in outcome-based rehabilitation, there are specific tools with which they must work in order to guide their behavior. Without the tools described here, staff may understand the concept but have difficulty changing their behavior toward an outcome-based model.

Tools for Outcome-Based Rehabilitation

1. A schema for defining clinical outcome: How is an outcome defined? What are the parameters? One example of a broad schema for identifying clinical outcomes has been developed by the Paradigm Corporation (see Exhibit 7–1).
2. A patient-centered assessment that crosses all disciplines: This approach to assessment allows the team to focus on functional skill areas, functional limitations, and how they impact disability. The focus of the assessment is on role resumption. From this assessment the treatment plan can be developed and treatment activities prioritized. Therapists may want to use portions of their discipline-based assessments to supplement the patient-centered assessment. Exhibit 7–2 is an example of an outcome plan based on an interdisciplinary patient-centered evaluation.
3. Critical pathways: Critical pathways are guidelines for mapping out the progression of treatment activities and the anticipated outcome within a specified time frame. The pathway should identify the time of team conference, time when family teaching will be initiated, and other programmatic components required to achieve the projected outcome. Another important component of a critical pathway is identifying accountability. Clinicians may be asked to sign the pathway to acknowledge that teaching of a particular skill has been completed and skill acquisition achieved. In this way the pathway may become a part of the patient's chart and can serve as documentation (see Exhibit 7–3).
4. A documentation system that is user-friendly and outcome-oriented: Documentation that is time consuming, is duplicative, and focuses on the patient's impairment status (e.g., balance, memory

Exhibit 7–1 Paradigm Rehabilitation Outcome Levels

Paradigm rehabilitation outcome levels are based on functional level of independence. Each outcome level requires the achievement or maintenance of all previous outcome levels. The outcome levels are defined below along with the patient's status: Achieved, In Progress, Targeted Outcome, Potential Future Outcome, and/or Not Clinically Feasible.

Level I   **Physiologic Medical Stability** – *Medical conditions diagnosed and stabilized and medical, nursing, nutritional and support protocols developed and in place to allow long-term management and remediation of medical and secondary complications.*

Level II   **Basic Rehabilitation Outcome** – *Limited level of functional independence in self-care, mobility, safety, and communication. Maximum level of assistance and supervision required.*

Level III   **Intermediate Rehabilitation Outcome** – *Moderate level of functional independence in self-care, mobility, safety, and communication. Moderate level of assistance and supervision required.*

Level IV   **Advanced Rehabilitation Outcome** – *Maximal level of functional independence in self-care, mobility, safety, communication, and home and community integration. Minimal level of assistance and supervision required.*

Level V   **Productive Activity** – *Fully integrated into productive activity including household management, school, and supported or nonsupported employment. Some assistance and supervision may be required.*

Source: Courtesy of Paradigm Health Corporation, Concord, California.

Exhibit 7–2 Premier Outcome Plan for Meeting Customer Goals and Expectations

Client Name: _____   Date of Admission: _____

Client Outcome Expectation(s):

Family Outcome Expectation(s):

Funder Outcome Expectation(s):

Physician Outcome Expectation(s):

Date Established or Date Revised	Agreed Upon Outcome Expectations	Projected Date for Completion	Discontinued	Revision Date	Achieved
	Projected Residential Goal: _____	_____	_____	_____	_____
_____		_____			
_____	*Revisions to Goal:* _____	_____			

Source: Reprinted from *Premier Outcome Plan for Meeting Customer Goals and Expectations* with Permission of Premier Rehabilitation, Inc., © 1994.

continues

Exhibit 7–2 continued

Page: _____

Client Name: _____

Date Established or Date Revised	Agreed Upon Outcome Expectations	Projected Date for Completion	Discontinued	Revision Date	Achieved
	Projected Productive Activity Goal:				
	Revisions to Goal:				
	Additional Outcome Goal:				
	Additional Outcome Goal				

Reviewed By Client: _____ Date: _____

Reviewed By Family: _____ Date: _____

Reviewed By Funder: _____ Date: _____

Reviewed By Physician: _____ Date: _____

Reviewed By Premier Case Manager: _____ Date: _____

continues

Exhibit 7–2 continued

Page: _____   Client Name: _____

Outcome Goal: _____
_____
_____

Attributes/Qualities/Characteristics which will assist in reaching this outcome goal: _____

Barriers to be overcome for the Client to be able to reach this outcome goal: _____

Measure # _____ to achieve goal: _____
_____   Date Estab. _____
_____   Projected Date _____
_____   Revision Date _____
_____   Date Achieved _____

Outcome Team Members Participating in Reaching this Measure:
___ Health Educator   ___ Speech & Language Pathologist   ___ Occupational Therapist   ___ Physical Therapist
___ Therapeutic Recreation Specialist   ___ Vocational Specialist   ___ Behavior Therapist   ___ Social Worker
Strategies/Objectives/Interventions to Reach this Measure   Staff Responsible   Proj. Date   Date Achieved

continues

Exhibit 7-2 continued

Page: _____

Client Name: _____

Measure # _____ to achieve goal:

_____

_____

_____

_____

Date Estab. _____
Projected Date _____
Revision Date _____
Date Achieved _____

Outcome Team Members Participating in Reaching this Measure:

___ Health Educator   ___ Speech & Language Pathologist   ___ Occupational Therapist   ___ Physical Therapist

___ Therapeutic Recreation Specialist   ___ Vocational Specialist   ___ Behavior Therapist   ___ Social Worker

Strategies/Objectives/Interventions to Reach this measure   Staff Responsible   Proj. Date   Date Achieved

Measure # _____ to achieve goal:

_____

_____

_____

_____

Date Estab. _____
Projected Date _____
Revision Date _____
Date Achieved _____

Outcome Team Members Participating in Reaching this Measure:

___ Health Educator   ___ Speech & Language Pathologist   ___ Occupational Therapist   ___ Physical Therapist

___ Therapeutic Recreation Specialist   ___ Vocational Specialist   ___ Behavior Therapist   ___ Social Worker

Strategies/Objectives/Interventions to Reach this measure   Staff Responsible   Proj. Date   Date Achieved

continues

Exhibit 7–2 continued

Page: _____   Client Name: _____

Measure # _____ to achieve goal:

_____   Date Estab. _____
_____   Projected Date _____
_____   Revision Date _____
_____   Date Achieved _____

Outcome Team Members Participating in Reaching this Measure:

___Health Educator   ___Speech & Language Pathologist   ___Occupational Therapist   ___Physical Therapist
___Therapeutic Recreation Specialist   ___Vocational Specialist   ___Behavior Therapist   ___Social Worker

Strategies/Objectives/Interventions to Reach this Measure   Staff Responsible   Proj. Date   Date Achieved

Measure # _____ to achieve goal:

_____   Date Estab. _____
_____   Projected Date _____
_____   Revision Date _____
_____   Date Achieved _____

Outcome Team Members Participating in Reaching this Measure:

___Health Educator   ___Speech & Language Pathologist   ___Occupational Therapist   ___Physical Therapist
___Therapeutic Recreation Specialist   ___Vocational Specialist   ___Behavior Therapist   ___Social Worker

Strategies/Objectives/Interventions to Reach this Measure   Staff Responsible   Proj. Date   Date Achieved

continues

Exhibit 7–2 continued

Premier Outcome Progress Report

Client Name: _____   Reporting Period: _____

Agreed Upon Outcome Expectation: _____

Measure to Accomplish Goal	Strategy Intervention to Accomplish Measure	Baseline Data	Progress/ Current Status	Plan for Next Reporting Period

Interpretation:

Therapist(s) Signature: _____ Date: _____   Date: _____
_____ Date: _____   Date: _____
_____ Date: _____   Date: _____

Client Signature: _____ Date: _____

Exhibit 7–3 AdvantageHEALTH/New England Rehabilitation Hospital Patient-Centered Rehabilitation Critical Pathway (PCRCP) [Young Stroke Program]

Program Documentation Form

I. Continuing Care Planning Process	First 72 Hours	Treatment Week 1	Treatment Week 2	Treatment Week 3	72 Hours Prior to Discharge
A. ADMISSION PROCESS AND CONSULT	Payer notified of patient's admission __/__/__ Physical Therapy __/__/__ Occupational Therapy __/__/__ Communication Disorders __/__/__ Neuropsychology __/__/__ Family Therapy __/__/__ Nutrition __/__/__ Consider Casting __/__/__ Consider Pool Therapy __/__/__ Neuropsychology __/__/__ Family Therapy __/__/__ Nutrition __/__/__ Vocational __/__/__	Wheelchair clinic __/__/__	Brace clinic __/__/__		
VARIANCE REPORT					

continues

Exhibit 7–3 continued

Program Documentation Form

	First 72 Hours	Treatment Week 1	Treatment Week 2	Treatment Week 3	72 Hours Prior to Discharge
I. Continuing Care Planning Process					
B. PROGRAM MONITOR-ING AND COORDINATION	Initial team meeting __/__/__ Family conference date established __/__/__	Team conference __/__/__	Team conference __/__/__ Family Teaching __/__/__	Team conference __/__/__ Family conference held __/__/__ Therapeutic pass scheduled __/__/__	
VARIANCE REPORT					
IV. Program Elements [FOCUS ON HOME SETTING]					
A. Mobility	Falls precautions screening __/__/__ PT evaluation completed __/__/__ PT/OT Nsg coordinate bed and wheelchair positioning, transfers, and activity on unit __/__/__ Up in chair __/__/__	Up in chair __/__/__ Wheelchair transfers to toilet; assisted wheelchair mobility in hallways __/__/__ Mobility training: Bed Mobility __/__/__ Transfers __/__/__	Up in chair __/__/__ Assisted ambulation in room __/__/__ Ambulatory transfers to toilet; wheelchair mobility in hallways __/__/__	Unsupervised ambulation in room __/__/__ Assisted ambulation in hallways __/__/__ Mobility training: Transfers __/__/__ Ambulation __/__/__	

continues

Exhibit 7–3 continued

Program Documentation Form

IV. **Program Elements** [FOCUS ON HOME SETTING]	First 72 Hours	Treatment Week 1	Treatment Week 2	Treatment Week 3	72 Hours Prior to Discharge
A. MOBILITY (cont.)	Assisted ambulation in room ___/___/___ Mobility training: Bed mobility ___/___/___ Transfers ___/___/___ Sitting balance ___/___/___ Assisted ambulation ___/___/___	Sitting balance ___/___/___ Assisted ambulation ___/___/___	Mobility training: Bed mobility ___/___/___ Transfers ___/___/___ Sitting balance ___/___/___ Assisted ambulation ___/___/___ Functional Mobility Group ___/___/___	Functional Mobility Group ___/___/___ Unsupervised ambulation in hallways ___/___/___ Gait Group ___/___/___	
CLINICAL INDICATORS					
VARIANCE REPORT					

continues

Exhibit 7-3 continued

168   OUTCOME-ORIENTED REHABILITATION

Program Documentation Form

IV. Program Elements [FOCUS ON HOME SETTING]	First 72 Hours	Treatment Week 1	Treatment Week 2	Treatment Week 3	72 Hours Prior to Discharge
MOBILITY OUTCOMES	Bed, chair, wheelchair transfer A: ___ LTG: ___ Locomotion -walk A: ___ Distance: ___ Device: ___ LTG: ___ Distance: ___ Device: ___ Locomotion -WC A: ___ Distance: ___ Device: ___ LTG: ___ Distance: ___ Device: ___ Stairs: A: ___ LTG: ___ # Steps ___ Device: ___ Sitting tolerance ___	Sitting tolerance ___ Bed, chair, wheelchair transfer C: ___ STG: ___ Locomotion -walk C: ___ Distance: ___ Device: ___ STG: ___ Distance: ___ Device: ___ Locomotion -WC C: ___ Distance: ___ Device: ___ STG: ___ Distance: ___ Device: ___ Stairs: C: ___ # Steps: ___ Device: ___ STG: ___ # Steps ___ Device: ___	Sitting tolerance ___ Bed, chair, wheelchair transfer C: ___ STG: ___ Locomotion -walk C: ___ Distance: ___ Device: ___ STG: ___ Distance: ___ Device: ___ Locomotion -WC C: ___ Distance: ___ Device: ___ STG: ___ Distance: ___ Device: ___ Stairs: C: ___ # Steps: ___ Device: ___ STG: ___ # Steps ___ Device: ___	Bed, chair, wheelchair transfer C: ___ STG: ___ Locomotion -walk C: ___ Distance: ___ Device: ___ STG: ___ Distance: ___ Device: ___ Locomotion -WC C: ___ Distance: ___ Device: ___ STG: ___ Distance: ___ Device: ___ Stairs: C: ___ # Steps: ___ Device: ___ STG: ___ # Steps ___ Device: ___	Bed, chair, wheelchair transfer D: ___ LTG: ___ Locomotion -walk LTG: ___ Distance: ___ Device: ___ D: ___ Distance: ___ Device: ___ Locomotion -WC LTG: ___ Distance: ___ Device: ___ D: ___ Distance: ___ Device: ___ Stairs: LTG: ___ # Steps: ___ Device: ___ D: ___ # Steps ___ Device: ___
MOBILITY OUTCOMES VARIANCE REPORT					

continues

Exhibit 7-3 continued

Program Documentation Form

IV. **Program Elements** [FOCUS ON HOME SETTING]	First 72 Hours	Treatment Week 1	Treatment Week 2	Treatment Week 3	72 Hours Prior to Discharge
B. PERSONAL CARE	OT/CD/Nsg coordinate feeding program __/__/__ CD evaluation of swallowing __/__ Determine need for upper extremity positioning device __/__ Feeding equipment evaluation __/__ Dressing evaluation __/__ Bathing evaluation at bed or sink level __/__	Young Stroke Group __/__ Feeding re-training __/__ Bathing and dressing re-training __/__ Assess adaptive equipment needs __/__	Young Stroke Group __/__ Grooming re-training __/__ Feeding re-training __/__ Bathing and dressing re-training __/__ Reassessed adaptive equipment needs __/__	Young Stroke Group __/__ Assess tub transfers and shower skills __/__ Assess equipment needs for tub/shower __/__ Grooming re-training __/__ Feeding re-training __/__ Bathing and dressing re-training __/__	
CLINICAL INDICATORS					
VARIANCE REPORT					

continues

Exhibit 7–3 continued

Program Documentation Form

IV. Program Elements [FOCUS ON HOME SETTING]	First 72 Hours	Treatment Week 1	Treatment Week 2	Treatment Week 3	72 Hours Prior to Discharge
PERSONAL CARE OUTCOMES	Eating A: ___ LTG: ___ Device: ___ Grooming A: ___ LTG: ___ Bathing A: ___ LTG: ___ Tub, Shower A: ___ LTG: ___ Device: ___ Dressing–Upper Body A: ___ LTG: ___ Dressing–Lower Body A: ___ LTG: ___	Eating C: ___ STG: ___ Device: ___ Grooming C: ___ STG: ___ Bathing C: ___ STG: ___ Tub, Shower C: ___ STG: ___ Device: ___ Dressing–Upper Body C: ___ STG: ___ Dressing–Lower Body C: ___ STG: ___	Eating C: ___ STG: ___ Device: ___ Grooming C: ___ STG: ___ Bathing C: ___ STG: ___ Tub, Shower C: ___ STG: ___ Device: ___ Dressing–Upper Body C: ___ STG: ___ Dressing–Lower Body C: ___ STG: ___	Eating C: ___ STG: ___ Device: ___ Grooming C: ___ STG: ___ Bathing C: ___ STG: ___ Tub, Shower C: ___ STG: ___ Device: ___ Dressing–Upper Body C: ___ STG: ___ Dressing–Lower Body C: ___ STG: ___	Eating C: ___ STG: ___ Device: ___ Grooming C: ___ STG: ___ Bathing C: ___ STG: ___ Tub, Shower C: ___ STG: ___ Device: ___ Dressing–Upper Body C: ___ STG: ___ Dressing–Lower Body C: ___ STG: ___
C. TOILETING	Nursing evaluation of bowel and bladder status ___/___ OT evaluation of clothes management and transfers ___/___				

continues

Exhibit 7-3 continued

Program Documentation Form

IV. Program Elements [FOCUS ON HOME SETTING]	First 72 Hours	Treatment Week 1	Treatment Week 2	Treatment Week 3	72 Hours Prior to Discharge
C. TOILETING (cont.) CLINICAL INDICATORS					
VARIANCE REPORT					
TOILETING OUTCOMES	Bladder Management A: ___ LTG: ___ Bowel Management A: ___ LTG: ___ Toilet transfers A: ___ LTG: ___ Device: ___	Bladder Management A: ___ LTG: ___ Bowel Management A: ___ LTG: ___ Toilet transfers A: ___ LTG: ___ Device: ___	Bladder Management A: ___ LTG: ___ Bowel Management A: ___ LTG: ___ Toilet transfers A: ___ LTG: ___ Device: ___	Bladder Management A: ___ LTG: ___ Bowel Management A: ___ LTG: ___ Toilet transfers A: ___ LTG: ___ Device: ___	Bladder Management A: ___ LTG: ___ Bowel Management A: ___ LTG: ___ Toilet transfers A: ___ LTG: ___ Device: ___
TOILETING OUTCOMES VARIANCE REPORT					

continues

Exhibit 7–3 continued

Program Documentation Form

IV. Program Elements [FOCUS ON HOME SETTING]	First 72 Hours	Treatment Week 1	Treatment Week 2	Treatment Week 3	72 Hours Prior to Discharge
D. HOME MANAGEMENT/SAFETY		CD Evaluation for home safety concerns ___/___/___ OT evaluation for home management ___/___/___		Assess meal preparation and planning skills ___/___/___ Assess living setting budgeting ___/___/___	
CLINICAL INDICATORS					
VARIANCE REPORT					
HOME MANAGEMENT OUTCOMES					
HOME MANAGEMENT VARIANCE REPORT					

continues

Exhibit 7–3 continued

Program Documentation Form

IV. Program Elements [FOCUS ON HOME SETTING]	First 72 Hours	Treatment Week 1	Treatment Week 2	Treatment Week 3	72 Hours Prior to Discharge
E. COMMUNICATION CLINICAL INDICATORS	CD Evaluation ___/___/___				
VARIANCE REPORT					
COMMUNICATION OUTCOMES	Comprehension Auditory A:___ LTG:___ Comprehension Visual A:___ LTG:___ Vocal Expression A:___ LTG:___ Nonvocal Expression A:___ LTG:___	Comprehension Auditory A:___ LTG:___ Comprehension Visual A:___ LTG:___ Vocal Expression A:___ LTG:___ Nonvocal Expression A:___ LTG:___	Comprehension Auditory A:___ LTG:___ Comprehension Visual A:___ LTG:___ Vocal Expression A:___ LTG:___ Nonvocal Expression A:___ LTG:___	Comprehension Auditory A:___ LTG:___ Comprehension Visual A:___ LTG:___ Vocal Expression A:___ LTG:___ Nonvocal Expression A:___ LTG:___	Comprehension Auditory A:___ LTG:___ Comprehension Visual A:___ LTG:___ Vocal Expression A:___ LTG:___ Nonvocal Expression A:___ LTG:___

continues

Exhibit 7-3 continued

Program Documentation Form

IV. Program Elements [FOCUS ON HOME SETTING]	First 72 Hours	Treatment Week 1	Treatment Week 2	Treatment Week 3	72 Hours Prior to Discharge
F. SOCIAL INTERACTION/ BEHAVIOR	NSG CD Evaluation/Screen __/__/__				Community resources established __/__/__
CLINICAL INDICATORS					
VARIANCE REPORT					
SOCIAL INTERACTION/ BEHAVIORAL OUTCOMES	Social Interaction A: ___ LTG: ___ Problem Solving A: ___ LTG: ___ Memory A: ___ LTG: ___	Social Interaction A: ___ LTG: ___ Problem Solving A: ___ LTG: ___ Memory A: ___ LTG: ___	Social Interaction A: ___ LTG: ___ Problem Solving A: ___ LTG: ___ Memory A: ___ LTG: ___	Social Interaction A: ___ LTG: ___ Problem Solving A: ___ LTG: ___ Memory A: ___ LTG: ___	Social Interaction A: ___ LTG: ___ Problem Solving A: ___ LTG: ___ Memory A: ___ LTG: ___
SOCIAL INTERACTION/ BEHAVIORAL OUTCOMES VARIANCE REPORT					

deficits, upper extremity strength) is not useful in an outcome-based model. This type of documentation fails to communicate progress toward the functional outcome. It also forces the therapist to focus on the impairment instead of reducing handicapping conditions. An outcome-based documentation system will be data-driven (McLean, Chapter 12) and will focus on functional skill requirements of the discharge environment.

5. An outcome tracking system: A longitudinal outcome tracking system is an essential tool for outcome-based rehabilitation. The process of deciding what outcome data will be collected, with what frequency, and by which collecting method is important. These decisions need to be made with team input because this process requires the team to select those outcomes they consider important. Organizations that assign this responsibility to the management information system department or to the "program evaluation people" are missing a valuable teaching opportunity for staff who are responsible for producing the outcome.

Outcome data provide the feedback teams need in order to know whether their intervention has been effective and whether the outcome will be durable. Outcome data allow program managers/directors to evaluate and modify clinical processes, resource utilization, and methods of interventions. Such data also become the basis for program evaluation. Often, team members do not understand the relationships among clinical outcomes, the outcome tracking system, and program evaluation. One of the best methods for giving team members accountability for clinical outcomes is to involve them in the decisions about selecting performance measures for evaluating outcomes and to educate them about the relationships of performance measures, outcome tracking, and program evaluation.

TEAM COMMUNICATION

Frequent and efficient communication among team members is essential in moving the team toward outcome-based rehabilitation. Teams may need to evaluate the "language" they use to describe goals, objectives, and outcomes. Language used to describe progress that is impairment-focused will create barriers for team discussions around outcome. Goals and objectives need to be stated in functional terms and must clearly address the outcome. Discipline-based goals that do not relate to the outcome are irrelevant in an outcome-based model. The team that is able to change its language from "discipline-oriented" and "limitation-focused" to "outcome-oriented" and "functionally focused" will be able to communicate effectively with one another and with their consumers.

The purpose and format of team conferences should also be evaluated. Within an outcome-based model, the purpose of a team conference is to provide information about patients' progress toward their outcome and to problem-solve barriers that may prevent sufficient movement toward the outcome. In a traditional service-based rehabilitation model, the purpose of a team conference is to provide the physician leader with a status update. Often the status update is discipline-based and focuses on impairments.

Example Dialog of Outcome-Based Team Conference

The case manager begins the discussion as follows:

In our initial team conference we projected the desired outcome from acute rehabilitation for Mrs. Jones as follows: return to her home with safety skills sufficient for her to be left alone without supervision for up to 4 hours each day. Her daughter will be able to assist her in her morning ADLs until she is able to be independent. She wants to be able to play bridge with her friends monthly as soon as possible. She is currently mildly depressed over her lack of independence and therefore we want to involve her in supportive counseling. We have anticipated a 2-week length of stay in which to accomplish her inpatient goals. Let's review her status and progress toward goals in the following areas:

- Mobility
- Health management
- Personal care
- Toileting
- Home management
- Emergency skills/safety
- Communication/social cognition
- Psychosocial/behavioral issues
- Patient/family teaching
- Outdoor mobility
- Community skills

- Recommendation for services needed to extend goals post discharge

The case manager asks for an update in each of the areas, and anyone who has been working with the patient in each area provides functionally relevant information. If barriers to outcome exist, the team has a problem-solving discussion using the following format:

- Emergency Skills
  - Objective: Mrs. Jones will use the medical alert call system independently.
  - Status: Mrs. Jones needs verbal cues and prompting to initiate.
  - Current barrier: Mrs. Jones does not believe she needs this system to access emergency care. She believes if she has an emergency her neighbor will be able to get help for her.
  - Next step to achieve objective: A home visit will occur whereby an emergency situation will be simulated. Mrs. Jones will be shown the steps of using the medical alert system as an alternative to calling her neighbor, in the event her neighbor is not home.

Example Dialog of a Service-Based Rehabilitation Team Conference

The physician begins the discussion:

Mrs. Jones has become medically stabilized. I am beginning to wean her off dilantin and am hoping this will help her to clear cognitively. She has swelling in the right knee due to a possible hematoma. I am continuing to monitor that. She complains of being depressed over her state of dependency. We have set goals for her to go home. Let's review how she is doing: Are there issues in nursing? How is she progressing in physical therapy, occupational therapy, etc.

At the conclusion social service or case management staff would be asked to comment on the status of the family and their adjustment. Case management or social service personnel would typically ask, "How long do you (the team) think Mrs. Jones will be here? The family wants to know."

Daily Progress Updates

In addition to regular team conferences that may occur weekly or every other week, the case manager will often need to check in with team members daily about patient progress. This daily communication may be organized into a daily stand-up meeting each morning for 15 minutes with the team for quick updates or problems that may have arisen, or the case manager may choose to go around to each team member and check in to gain daily updates. The daily stand-up meeting time is best utilized when the team has progress data in the form of graphs/charts that allow for an objective review of daily change (Figures 7–1 and 7–2). Many facilities are reluctant to allow daily team meetings. As long as they are kept to a minimum of 15 to 30 minutes, this daily team communication allows everyone on the team to be updated simultaneously and is not more time consuming than individually updating the case manager on each patient. Regardless of the form it takes, daily communication around patient status and progress to the outcome is vital as length of stay decreases and accountability for outcome is heightened.

TEACHING STAFF TO WORK WITH FAMILIES WITHIN AN OUTCOME-BASED MODEL

Outcome goals and objective around family adjustment, family training, and long-term consequences of the disability should be integral components of the overall rehabilitation plan. Family outcome goals should be developed and monitored for achievement just as patient outcome goals are monitored. Exhibit 7–4 identifies outcome goals and objectives with which families may be involved.

In addition to working with families on their outcomes, staff need to work hand in hand with families on the patient's outcome. Facilitating goals for the patient's outcome using family involvement while assisting family goal attainment can be difficult.

Shifting to an outcome-based model from the perspective of working with families will be more difficult for staff who have previously functioned from an "expert-driven model." Within an expert model staff see themselves as the experts who provide information to the family. Within the model, the families' role is to receive information, ask questions, and adjust. This role is limiting for families and for the team.

In an outcome-based model, the staff work in a consultative role with the family.

Exhibit 7–4 Family Outcomes

Family Disability Adjustment

The objective of the family disability adjustment outcome is to facilitate the initiation of resumption of individual family member life roles through coordinated education and counseling by appropriate professionals and treatment team members.

The spouse/parents/siblings/significant others may be able to demonstrate the initiation of resumption of their personal life roles that include

- returning to a reasonable work schedule
- returning to community activities
- attending to the needs of noninjured family members
- sustaining and maintaining social relationships
- obtaining adequate rest
- engaging in leisure activities
- returning to a balanced schedule
- attending to own personal needs
- allowing (patient) autonomy

Family Issue Identification

The objective of this outcome is to identify family concerns and issues relative to the patient and his or her injury and handicap that may impact on long-term function and management through assessments by appropriate professionals.

Family Training for the Home

The objective of this outcome is to educate and train the patient's family and care providers relative to management of the patient in the home environment, including cognitive/behavioral/safety/communication/self-care/mobility strategies that allow for optimal autonomy of the patient.

Family Training for the Community

The objective of this outcome is to educate and train the patient's family and care provider relative to management of the patient in the community environment, including cognitive/behavioral/communication/safety/mobility strategies that allow for optimal autonomy of the patient.

Source: Courtesy of Paradigm Health Corporation, Concord, California.

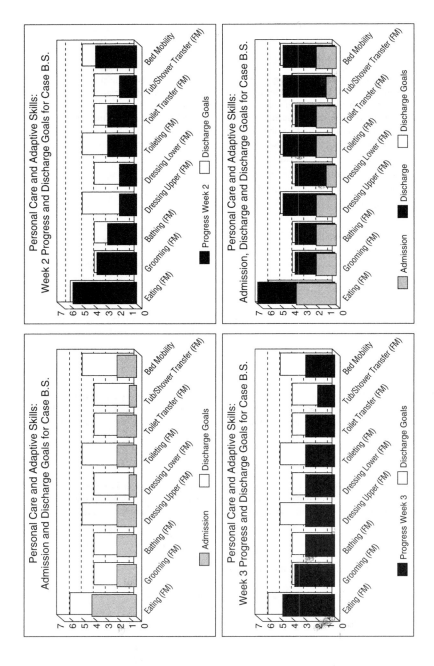

Figure 7-1 Summary of Functional Progress for Case B.S.—Personal Care and Adaptive Skills

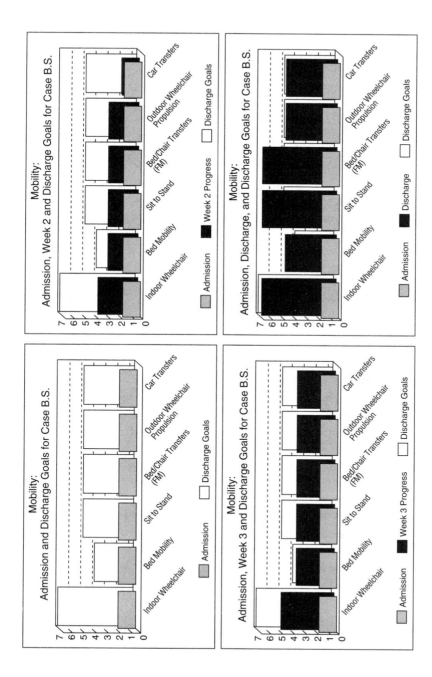

Figure 7-2 Summary of Functional Progress for Case B.S.—Mobility

- They determine together what the family needs to be able to take their family member home. Families should be asked by the staff, "What is the most important skill your family member needs to acquire for you to be able to manage your relative within the home setting?"
- Staff teach the family skills the patient needs to be able to do in the home. In many cases the family will be given a care plan to implement in the home. Teaching the family this care plan will begin within the first 2 weeks of the rehabilitation program. The family and the staff will collaborate and alter the care plan according to feedback from the family.
- The family will make adjustments to the disability of their injured relative. The impact of the disability on the family should be discussed and appropriate outcome goals established.

Working with the family in a consultative mode requires the staff and the family to interact constantly. Family participation in the rehabilitation program must be active and occur on a daily basis in order for the desired outcome to be achieved. The expectation that families will need to be actively involved in the rehabilitation of their loved one should be discussed prior to admission. When families are not able to participate, for reasons such as lack of transportation or child care, the expectation for outcome must be adjusted accordingly.

It is important that staff see themselves as consultants to the family, and, like any good consultants, they should work themselves out of a job. The staff want the family to succeed in returning their family member to the home environment. In order for the family to succeed, they need to be trained on how to cue their family member and how to provide appropriate assistance in order to facilitate optimal independence.

Shifting into a consultative model may require role playing and rehearsal to allow staff to be successful in this approach. A family therapist or social worker who has been trained in a consultative approach to working with families is a key individual to help staff move into this model of interaction.

Family Counseling

Working with families toward outcome achievement will be most successful when families are assisted with their emotional adjustment to their loved one's disability through appropriate family counseling.

Family counseling and family teaching should remain separate in the way they are provided to the family. Family teaching may elicit emotional reactions by families, and staff should be trained on how to assist them through this reaction. A common reaction of families, for example, is resistance to family teaching. A family member may cancel family teaching appointments, miss appointments, or be unavailable. One possible response to this situation is to develop a contract with the family in which expectations of the family and team are clearly defined. A contract like this will work best when initiated by the case manager, not the family therapist. While the family therapist and case manager work hand in hand, their roles in interacting with the family are distinct.

Family counseling is vital to outcome achievement by the family. It is important to distinguish family therapy or counseling from family education and family teaching. Both contribute to the overall outcome of the patient and family but should be accessed by the family in distinctly separate ways.

Staff Support Group

Providing a support group is vital for rehabilitation staff. The purpose of the support group is to provide a forum for staff to talk of their feeling about their work.[1] Moving from traditional service-based rehabilitation to outcome-based rehabilitation is a shift that creates many feelings within staff. Through an appropriately led support group, staff have the opportunity to air their feelings and constructively work through these issues. Some of the issues that staff struggle with when moving into an outcome-based model are as follows:

- We can't predict an outcome when we don't know how the patient will respond to treatment.
- This approach forces us to work on only a few areas; we should work on all areas that need to be addressed.
- We don't have enough time to do the work for which we were trained. If we had more time, we could do a better job.
- We want rehabilitation to be the way it used to be, when we could take our time and really get to know the patients and families.
- We went into rehabilitation to help "restore independence" for our patients; now we work on only a piece of that goal.
- This is not the way we were trained to work (therefore, it is not valid).

The feelings that are associated with these issues include feelings of loss, anger, anxiety, and frustration. Many times staff may be mourning the "way things used to be." They may also feel guilty and inadequate for not being able to give patients more services, assuming that "more is better." In addition, most individuals resist change. Moving into an outcome-based model creates tremendous change for staff, and feelings associated with this change must have a forum in which to be addressed.

In addition to staff experiencing feelings of loss, anger, anxiety, and mourning about their work situation, patients and families are also experiencing these same feelings. This situation sets up a scenario described by Gans as "hate in the rehabilitation setting."[2] If these feelings are not acknowledged and clarified for staff, they will be played out in the rehabilitation workplace. When this happens, feelings may be inappropriately displaced on other staff, administration, even patients and their families. A staff support group will provide an opportunity to name these feelings and work through them.

CONCLUSION

The goal of this chapter was to outline the various steps involved in moving interdisciplinary teams toward an outcome-based model of rehabilitation. Four steps were outlined.

1. Leading and managing the organization from an outcome perspective
2. Providing senior management support for interdisciplinary teams toward outcome-based rehabilitation
3. Organizing and training staff for outcome-based rehabilitation
4. Teaching staff to work with families from an outcome-based perspective

Each of these steps must be conceptualized and implemented in a systematic manner for outcome-based rehabilitation to be a "positive outcome" for the people we serve, our staff, and the organization.

In addition to the organization following the broad systematic steps outlined, rehabilitation teams who provide outcome-based rehabilitation will complete the following ten steps for outcome achievement with their patients and families.

1. Determine the outcome(s)/result to be achieved.
2. Obtain consensus from the patient, family, and rehabilitation team of the outcome.

3. Assess to determine baseline in relation to the target level of functioning needed to achieve the outcome.

4. Determine the critical pathway for achieving the outcome.

5. Train to the criterion necessary to achieve the outcome.

6. Measure progress against the critical path milestones.

7. Determine whether milestones are being achieved. If they are, outcome achievement is on target.

8. Make one of two choices if the milestones are not being met.

   a. Readjust the time frame for achieving the milestones and proceed on course at a different rate.

   b. Determine why you are off target and then make alterations in the outcome or in the strategy for achieving the outcome.

9. Obtain secondary confirmation that the criterion that is necessary to achieve the outcome has been met.

10. Celebrate the successful achievement of the outcome and establish an outcome stabilization procedure to assure that the outcome is being maintained. In most instances this will only involve monitoring, but no active interventions.

Moving toward outcome-based rehabilitation within the structure outlined in this chapter will allow the organization to make the necessary transition without losing staff or negatively impacting quality of care. It is critical that staff become part of this change process and not just recipients of it. Following the principles and steps outlined will help rehabilitation leaders and managers to be effective in preparing staff to move toward outcome-based rehabilitation.

REFERENCES

1. Ratner J, McNamara M. Staff support groups. *Hospital News and Healthcare Review.* 1994;3(8):12–18.

2. Gans JS. Hate in the rehabilitation setting. *Arch Phys Med Rehabil.* 1983;64:176–179.

Part II

Business Principles in Outcome-Focused Rehabilitation

The purpose of Part II is to articulate and apply principles of business excellence that enable an enterprise to deliver on their commitments to rehabilitation results.

Chapter 8

Designing the Enterprise for Outcome-Based Rehabilitation

John O'Lear, MBA

Objectives

- To address key issues associated with leading and managing an outcome-based rehabilitation enterprise.
- To provide specific suggestions for designing an outcome-based organization.
- To address front-end decision making regarding objectives, mission, definition, and strategy.
- To present the road map or operational plan for an outcome-based rehabilitation enterprise.

INTRODUCTION

In this chapter, the author will discuss the many issues associated with leading and managing an outcome-based rehabilitation enterprise. It is the author's intent to provide specific suggestions for designing and managing an outcome-based organization. These suggestions are applicable for not-for-profit organizations that expect to cover all costs and post some positive reserves, and for-profit organizations that expect to cover all costs including a return on investment for their shareholders. In either case, the leaders of the organization must explicitly determine the founding objectives, define the mission of the enterprise, raise resources to achieve that mission, and control those resources to produce value that exceeds the cost of providing services.

There will be considerable emphasis on front-end decision making, that is, decisions about the objectives of the enterprise, the definition, mission, and strategy. These elements refer to the strategic direction of the enterprise. These front-end decisions are very difficult to make but are the ones that provide the greatest leverage. After those decisions are made, however, the road map for execution becomes very important. It will be discussed as the operational plan. The subsections will analyze the objectives, background, definition, mission, vision, strategy, values, goals, performance measurements, and audit of the enterprise, as discussed in the material that follows.

Objectives of the Enterprise

Simply, why was the enterprise created? Since all other choices flow naturally from this single source it is very important to be clear and honest. If an organization was created to build assets for the stockholders, this objective should be made clear. This objective may be obtained while being a service to the community and acting as a responsible and ethical organization. The moral character of an enterprise is not defined by its objective but by the values espoused and followed by the organization. Organizations that define their objective not as building value for investors but as providing service to the community are as capable of corrupt and unethical behavior as those who define the objective as creating a return for stockholders. All other items to follow must be measured against these objectives.

Where Are We?

Background information must be collected to inform the planners about their environment.

Definition of the Enterprise

Defining the enterprise includes what is to be done for whom and where. The definition should be in very clear and concise language and reflect the enterprise customer's needs. Considerable thought is required to identify both the customer and the customer's needs. Many organizations leave this important step out of their policy planning or are vague and ambiguous, deciding, in essence by default, to do everything for everybody, everywhere. Focus is essential in designing the enterprise.

Mission of the Enterprise

What will be the result of the enterprise's work? It is easy to confuse mission and objective. The *mission* defines the results expected in clear, measurable terms. These terms may be expressed in measures such as market share, customer satisfaction, return on investment, and clinical outcomes. The mission statement may include various measures as long as they are not mutually exclusive. During the past decade, using vague and lofty mission statements has been in vogue. This practice may be impressive in the organization's marketing materials, but it does not serve the wider purpose of focusing all participants on what needs to be accomplished in order to fulfill the mission of the enterprise and accomplish the founding objectives.

Vision of the Enterprise

The vision of the enterprise is the result of looking ahead to determine the future on the basis of the accomplishment of the basic mission. The vision is what the enterprise will look like in the future; it inspires participants to accomplish the current mission and provides insight into current decisions concerning definition and mission.

Strategy

The enterprise will only accomplish its mission and fulfill its vision when value is produced for patients, payers, and employees that exceeds the cost of production. The main strategy of the enterprise indicates key decisions that determine how that will be accomplished.

Values of the Enterprise

What are the rules of play? This portion will deal with the importance of choosing and communicating culture and protocols for interpersonal communications and other processes and interactions. Selecting values and taking action consistent with those values determine the ethical nature of the enterprise.

Goals of the Enterprise

What are the specific operational targets and who will be accountable for achieving them? What is the process for setting priorities? How will opportunities and challenges be declared?

Performance Measurements

How will the enterprise know whether it is hitting the targets? This section will deal with specific tools for performance measurement based on continuous quality improvement in a clinical environment.

Audit of the Enterprise

Are we fulfilling our mission? This portion deals with periodic review to determine whether previous priorities and decisions are working, and, if so, whether they are bringing satisfaction to the patient, payer, and employees. Do the results suggest additional opportunity?

It is important to note that the process for designing the enterprise is iterative. Frequently, the definition of the enterprise may change as a result of conclusions reached during goal setting exercises. A different vision may alter the current mission statement. This process should be dynamic and ongoing. However, at all times, the various aspects of the enterprise should be in alignment and consistent in order to bring clarity and energy to the participant's efforts.

STRATEGIC PLAN

Objective of the Enterprise

Choosing clear objectives for the enterprise and documenting them in easy to understand language have a profound impact on the future success of the enterprise. All other choices made by the directors, managers, and employees should flow naturally from these decisions. It is important to note that an enterprise may offer individuals an opportunity to fulfill their objectives, which may by their nature be quite different from the objectives of the enterprise. For example, the enterprise may hire a researcher to carry out specific research that will contribute to the objectives of the enterprise and simultaneously advance the individual objectives of the researcher. The enterprise, however, must be careful to ensure that the objectives of the individual participants are consistent with the objectives and values of the enterprise.

The objective for the enterprise should be clearly stated by its founders when the enterprise is formed. If this is not the case, then efforts should be made to determine the implicit or explicit objective of the current shareholders or directors. The usual choices are to increase shareholder wealth or to provide a specific societal benefit. It is important to note that these are not mutually exclusive goals. There may be times, however, when the enterprise must make decisions on various aspects of the enterprise that will require selecting between two mutually exclusive actions. It is at these times that the decision makers must look to the founding objectives of the enterprise for guidance. Frequently, organizations are founded without objectives being explicitly stated or recorded. Often, even when explicitly stated, they have such sweeping and ambiguous language that they provide little guidance when managers of the enterprise consult them for decisions. In cases like this, phrases such as "That's all well and good, but we must remember that we have to answer to our shareholders," are frequently heard. This statement, of course, begs the question, What do the shareholders expect?

There are other choices that are based on the personal goals of the founders, which again should be clearly stated. Declaring the objectives of the enterprise, that is, stating clearly why the enterprise exists, should not be confused with the values by which the enterprise will operate. The objectives are not moral choices, but rather the legitimate decisions of those who work to create an enterprise. To declare that an enterprise exists solely to provide needed care to patients is a noble founding objective. But if in the course of carrying out the activities of the enterprise, other issues transcend this objective, the founding objective has failed to provide appropriate guidance to the managers. The intention of declaring only noble-sounding objectives results in confusion and disappointment among the participants, unless the objectives have been chosen honestly with full recognition of the consequences of those decisions.

Where Are We?

Before the planning process begins, it is important to collect specific information about the environment in which the enterprise exists. The following questions provide a checklist for those items:
- After determining the founding objectives, it is important to determine the personal objectives, as they apply to the design and implementation of the enterprise, of the key participants. These personal objectives will have profound influences on the enterprise.
- As an organization, given the founding objectives, what are the strengths and weaknesses of the enterprise?
- What are the needs, concerns, and desires of our anticipated customers?
- Who will be competing with the enterprise and what will their behavior likely be in the future?
- What do we need to understand about the demographics of the potential catchment areas?
- How will the health care and workers' compensation industry be structured in the future?

Definition of the Enterprise

The definition of the enterprise simply determines what the enterprise will do, for whom, and where. In order to be useful for decision making, this must be done from the customer's point of view. Obviously, defining the business in this manner suggests that the enterprise has a clear understanding of how the customer perceives its services. The importance of the definition of the enterprise cannot be overstated. Decisions on what services to offer and what markets and customers to serve have profound consequences to the long-term viability of any organization. Frequently, these decisions are so difficult that they are avoided or are worded so ambiguously that they provide little direction to the participants.

The following list indicates some of the issues to consider when selecting a definition:
- Review of possible diagnoses
- Review of potential services to offer
- Review of optional programs
- Review of payer groups

- Review of patient groups
- Review of catchment area

This exercise provides an opportunity for a thorough and thoughtful review to determine what the enterprise should do and for whom. It is important to understand that the resources for developing and executing the chosen areas must be identified in order to choose wisely. If a fully explicated pro forma detailing the resources required to develop and maintain a high degree of capability in the different areas is not developed, then the definition will generally suggest that the organization will do everything for everyone, anywhere. This approach obviously is not useful in designing an enterprise. It is also important to understand the role of other organizations, in the same or similar catchment areas, that offer similar services. Just committing to be the best will not result in a clear differentiation in the marketplace. Excess capacity of products and services in any area inevitably leads to low differentiation and ultimately to commodity pricing, which reduces margins below cost. On the other hand, offering services that are generally unavailable or underserved provides substantial opportunities for products and services that can be priced to exceed the full cost, allowing surpluses that can be used to improve service delivery, raise quality, and lower costs.

Detailed consideration of the possible combinations of products and services, markets to be served, and catchment area saves considerable time and prevents developing costly services that have no market demand.

Developing the list of possibilities is an exciting process. Providing detailed and intense review of these possibilities is laborious and tedious. The real payoff, however, comes from having done the homework required to choose the enterprise's definition carefully. One should spend 20 percent of the time creating possibilities and 80 percent of the time turning those possibilities into a well-defined enterprise that meets real customers' needs.

Mission of the Enterprise

After the business definition is complete, managers and their advisers can begin the process of establishing the mission of the enterprise. The specific definition of the mission statement as used in this text is not in accordance with the term as it is generally used. The term *mission statement,* as popularly used, refers to a statement of intended purpose of the organization and is usually described in platitudes about "serving our customers better." While these statements may provide spiritual inspiration to the participants and the intended customers, they generate more heat than light on what the enterprise is trying to accomplish. The definition, as used in this text, refers to those central goals that the enterprise should strive to achieve over an extended period, 3 to 5 years, in order to meet the founding objectives and fulfill the founding vision of the enterprise.

The mission of the organization defines the expected results to be obtained over a period. Generally, periods such as 3 to 5 years are chosen. An example: XYZ Enterprise will be the market share leader in x market, have customer satisfaction ratings exceeding 95 percent, have outcomes rated in the top quartile of the country, operate at a 20 percent return on equity, and be achieving a 15 percent annual growth in earnings. This mission statement sets forth market share goals, customer service goals, outcome achievement goals, and financial and growth goals. Each of the areas can be measured, allowing all participants to be informed periodically of how the enterprise is doing against its chosen mission statement.

Depending on the nature of the enterprise, during any given period, some of the goals in the preceding mission statement may be inappropriate. For example, in the early stages of an enterprise, having specific long-term (beyond 1 year) return on equity goals may be inappropriate. During this period, perhaps growth in revenues, customer satisfaction, and outcome achievement would provide focus and clarity to the organization. Specific annual budgets could be used to provide appropriate boundaries for utilizing resources to accomplish the mission.

Since the activities of the enterprise should be guided by the goals as stated in the mission statement, it is very important to think through the elements of the statement carefully. A well-developed mission statement, generally one paragraph in length, does not reflect the work that went into preparing such a statement. The quality of the mission statement, as measured by its usefulness to the enterprise over time, is determined by the quality of the thinking that went into the enterprise objectives, vision, definition, and goals. Again, it is important to consider this process as an iterative approach. Iteration is very important as the mission statement is defined. A careful review of previous elements and thinking, as well as drafting of some detailed pro formas to test the reasonableness of selected goals, is very important. A mission statement that is beyond the resources of the enterprise is very demoralizing to the participants and will result in a lack of commitment to the enterprise's mission.

Equally, mission statements that are vague and provide little useful guidance to the participants will act to undermine the commitment to the enterprise. The mission statement should not be a dream (dreams are better stated in the vision of the enterprise); rather it should be concrete, well thought out, and tested with pro forma models based on empirical data.

When market share goals are stated, they should be based on a clear understanding of the current market trends that will impact the future market and current and anticipated actions of competitors. While perfect information is never available, and even near-perfect information would be prohibitively expensive, practical information backed by careful analytical thought will provide sufficient direction to choose goals that will be useful in guiding the decisions of the enterprise. A discussion of market research is outside the scope of this chapter. It is important, however, to understand that one of the crucial decisions for costly market research is what the enterprise will do with the information. How will the answers be used, and is it possible that informed estimates may provide as much value as lengthy, costly, and uncertain searches for the "Holy Grail"?

When using goals based on subjective ratings, such as customer service, it is not necessary to answer questions about when or how these surveys will be conducted. That can be determined later. It is vital to consider the importance of the chosen area on the objectives of the enterprise and the long-term vision. For example, it is generally thought that good customer service is always important, but some enterprises have captured large market shares based on the importance of price and have avoided and even made a culture of avoiding normal or expected customer service requirements, so that lower prices could be offered. The importance of avoiding platitudes and carefully testing assumptions cannot be overstated.

The use of financial goals is as important for the nonprofit sector as for the for-profit sector. Actually, in terms of financial performance there is little difference between the two types of organizations other than tax status. In order to have long-term financial viability, the nonprofit organization must have revenues that exceed costs, resulting in an accumulation of surpluses much the same as in a for-profit organization. These surpluses are then used for longer-term investments and for working capital for growth.

The most difficult issue frequently encountered in setting financial goals is determining how realistic they are relative to market conditions and the other nonfinancial goals of the enterprise. If the financial health of the enterprise is at all threatened, the financial goals must take precedent over all other issues. In some cases, financial issues may be so severe that the only mission of the enterprise is the financial viability for the long term, subordinating all other issues until that situation is resolved. Any organization that focuses on a multitude of issues when severe cash flow problems exist or insolvency threatens is courting disaster. It is very difficult to take corrective action and to sacrifice short-term market position or other important aspects of the enterprise, but without strong, well-focused action, the enterprise may not survive.

What are appropriate financial goals to be included in the mission statement or provide boundaries for other goals stated in the mission statement? The financial goals should be stated in terms of return-on-investment measures, as opposed to profit as percentage of revenues. Profit percentages vary widely and say little about the overall financial health of the enterprise. Return-on-investment measures, such as return on equity or return on assets employed, are less volatile and provide a better measure of the financial aspects of the enterprise.

The final question of the usefulness of a specific mission statement is, If we accomplish the goals stated in the mission statement, are we assured that the objectives of the enterprise are being met, and, further, is the enterprise in a position to complete its vision for the long term? This test, of course, must be balanced by another test: How realistic are the goals specified in the mission statement? If the answer to both of these questions is positive, then the chosen mission statement should serve its intended purpose well.

Vision of the Enterprise

Generally when an enterprise is created, a vision exists that has guided the creative process. In addition, various objectives are probably understood if not clearly stated. The vision of the founders, however, may not be very precise or even useful to plan and govern the activities of the organization. If there is more than one founder, more than one vision may exist, but not be clearly understood. The value of creating a specific documented vision is that it provides a benchmark from which to measure how the organization is doing and to determine the correct goals for the future. Also, members of the enterprise can see more clearly what the results of accomplishing the organization's mission will mean.

While the vision of the organization can be stated in generalities, it should be concise and very clear. Equally important is the fact that the vision should include the customers, influences, and employees, and how they will benefit by having the enterprise succeed. The vision of the organization may be created by a single founding member or by many different members. In either case, it is very important to all members that the vision be consistent with the needs of the customers now and in the future, and that it be clearly, consistently, and frequently communicated.

Strategy of the Enterprise

Some of the most important elements in developing a comprehensive strategy for any enterprise have already been discussed in the definition of the enterprise: what will the enterprise do, for whom will it be done, and where will it be done. These decisions go a long way toward defining strategy. However, the issue of how it will be done and how the products and services will be positioned, packaged, and priced must be carefully addressed.

The Shouldice hospital, located just outside Toronto, Ontario, provides an excellent example of a well-chosen, integrated strategy for providing health care services. In its field, the Shouldice hospital is one of the most profitable facilities anywhere in the world, yet the hospital prices its service offerings at a fraction of the normal and customary charges of other institutions, both profit and nonprofit. In addition, the hospital has outstanding patient ratings and medical outcomes. How can this be? Shouldice has chosen to provide outstanding service for only one type of medical problem: the inguinal hernia. Patients come from around the world because of the hospital's reputation and outstanding outcomes. Frequently, major cost of travel is more than offset by the large difference in price between conventional centers and Shouldice. This success is an outstanding example of the power of centers of excellence when a specific strategy has been chosen.

The strategy employed by Shouldice hospital is based on technological development, specialization, and patient involvement in the recovery process. The technology employed is simply to screen patients carefully so that only those who are not otherwise ill are accepted for service. This screening procedure allows the use of local anesthetics, thereby preventing complications and the slower recovery process associated with general anesthetics. In addition, a special suture technique is used that promotes more rapid healing of the incision. The hospital rooms are spartan, and all luxuries, such as showers, telephones, and television, are available, but only after walking some distance to reach them. This layout not only reduces facility cost but, more important, encourages the patient to get exercise that facilitates rapid recovery.

The success of Shouldice has been realized by a strategic vision that incorporates planning elements that permit careful procedures that are targeted at reducing length of stay, maximizing service load, and reducing staff to be developed. For example, patients who have recently returned from surgery provide patient orientation for incoming patients at bedtime functions called "tea and cookies." While the strategy of Shouldice hospital is very creative, it is important to note that the process of creativity has been driven by the strategic choices made by the leadership of the hospital. Most organizations have unused creative capacity. What they lack is an environment and structure that will unleash this creativity to improve service delivery, quality, and productivity.

The example described incorporates many elements of the strategic process. What will we do, for whom will we do it, what will be the catchment area, and how will we do it better and faster? The hospital planning group did not count on being able to hire better people who would work harder for less money than their competitors. In fact, they realized that it was important to have employees who were happy in their respective roles and designed systems that would assure, with proper screening, that each doctor, nurse, and staff employee would have an opportunity to be fully productive and satisfied with the work.

The enterprise that chooses to provide rehabilitation services must carefully examine many issues to determine an appropriate strategy that will ensure good patient outcomes, good value to the payer and the patient, successful and happy employees, and economic viability. The starting point should be the examination of market segments. As in the example, patients who were otherwise healthy with the diagnosis of inguinal hernia and located anywhere in the world was the market segment chosen. Segments can be examined in terms of diagnostic groups, demographics, payer type, psychographics, and many more factors. Then, it is important to determine the specific needs of each segment and how well these needs are currently being served.

After a thorough analysis of alternative market segments, a position statement that details several optional service models should be drafted. Each service model considered should explicate how existing services are provided, how these services are priced, and how they could be provided more effectively and/or efficiently. A value-added model should be developed that specifically states the service level that will be provided and how that level will be valued by the payer and the patient.

An analysis that addresses each component of the proposed delivery system should then be performed. Ask the question, How can this be done differently to add greater value and/or decrease cost? The areas to consider are pricing terms, for example, episodic, per diem, and capitation; marketing systems; operating procedures; staffing; information systems; productivity; and quality. These areas and others may offer opportunities to differentiate the products and services being considered. From this examination, options may be chosen and then carefully described as customer specifications, similar to those found in most requests for proposals. These should then be tested by the use of various focus groups and one-on-one interviews. While this process seems laborious, the information and insight gained during it will prove valuable when final decisions are made and implementation plans are formed.

The process of analysis and synthesis for finding and adopting a strategy for the enterprise is work that is really never complete. The process must be circular and done over and over, refining existing strategies as well as defining new possibilities. When confronted with the challenge of creating value that exceeds the cost of production, strategic options are the most fertile ground for solutions.

Selecting the Values of the Enterprise

Most organizations have well-established value systems that inform all participants about the rules of play. These value systems may be the result of careful thought and planning, or they may be derived from the day-to-day behaviors of the participants. In either case, they have a profound influence on the success of the enterprise. It is important to note that if there are clearly declared values for the enterprise, it is imperative that behavior of management and staff conform to those stated values. This behavior is frequently referred to as "walking the talk."

When considering values that can be adopted, it is important to compare each with the other aspects of the enterprise, such as strategy, markets served, and founding objectives. The values selected should be internally consistent with the other choices. If they are not, major problems may develop and be difficult to understand and resolve. For example, if the enterprise states that it values creativity, but selects a strategy that is based on very strict adherence to step-by-step procedures and allows little latitude for change, creativity may be stifled, producing an atmosphere of hypocrisy.

There are special considerations to be made when establishing values in an outcome-based rehabilitation organization. Since the service model is fundamentally based on an interdisciplinary process, collaboration in determining values for the enterprise is very important. In addition, the values selected should reflect, and be consistent with, the best standards of practice for an interdisciplinary model.

The considerations made in selecting values for the enterprise should include the importance of ethics in the design and delivery of health care products and services. While there are many heated discussions in today's health care environment about the ethics of responsibility, medicine in general has had a 2,500-year history of a workable system of ethical guidelines as reflected in the Hippocratic oath given by the Greek physician: *Primum non nocere,* "Above all, not knowingly to do harm." There are many areas where both clinical and administrative managers are not always aware of the importance of these words. The role of all individuals in a health care system is to be sure that they do not knowingly do harm.

OPERATING PLAN

Priorities of the Enterprise

The previous material has set a strategic stage on which a well-selected cast of characters must execute a script that has only been defined in general terms. The next step is to create an operations plan that will serve as a detailed script that describes the characters, their roles and responsibilities, stage action, and the expected flow from beginning to end. This operations plan is the detailed blueprint for executing the mission of the enterprise. As such, it should be thorough, carefully developed, and internally consistent and form a complete bridge to the strategic plan. Does this mean that it must in all cases be correct? No! Plans at this stage are rarely "correct" and sufficient to accomplish the intended results. If it has been rigorously developed, however, any shortcomings should be noted quickly, and since the plan is a living document, it can be altered to address the identified weaknesses. The fact that plans are rarely correct does not suggest that one skip the detailed plans. The planning process alone will raise many questions, which may otherwise remain hidden until some very inopportune time then surface, creating chaos.

The operations plan details what needs to be done, who is accountable for doing it, when it should be completed, and what it will look like when it is completed (the deliverable). The first step to developing an effective operating plan is to identify the essential factors that are required to implement the strategy of the enterprise. Generally, these factors include a communications strategy for informing the patients and payers of the enterprise's capabilities and benefits; a detailed plan for service delivery, including critical pathways and protocols; and a financial model that quantifies all aspects of operations to assure appropriate margins.

Once these factors have been identified, assign appropriate personnel to draft detailed action plans describing the intended result of the action, how that result supports the mission of the enterprise, what the tasks are, and when and by whom they will be completed. When the results have been completed by the individuals assigned, a thorough and comprehensive review can be conducted by the interdisciplinary team who have assembled the various components. This step is very important since it offers considerable opportunity to integrate the organization and to be creative in planning and using resources. It is during this process that substantial information and insight into the actual functioning of the enterprise arise. For that reason, it is very important to consider the iterative nature of the planning process. Go back and review the strategic portions of the plan. Perhaps assumptions made during the strategic planning are being questioned during the development of the operations plan. If so, avoid trying to force fit the answers because of tight time lines or other organizational reasons. If the assumptions do not fit the planning realities, think about changing the assumptions. Also, look for other possibilities that have been raised during the development of the detailed plan. Remember that both God and the Devil can be in the detail.

During the process of developing detailed operating plans, it is very important to put numbers to every assumption and action plan. For example, if there is a discussion of developing an internal database that will demonstrate the clinical efficacy of selected critical pathways, be prepared to define the cost of designing, implementing, and maintaining the database. Then compare those costs to the expected incremental income, after covering costs for service delivery, that would be produced by sharing the data with payers and/or patients. Vary the estimates to determine the cost benefit from taking the planned action. Avoid assuming that because everyone thinks it's a good thing to do, it must be right.

Since numbers are generally thought to be a part of accounting and finance, there is a general tendency only to address these issues in the detailed financial pro formas. This practice is risky business. The accounting and finance function may play back the assumptions made, rather than evaluate the data for reasonableness and cost-effectiveness. Everyone involved with the planning process should be involved in the creation of assumptions and quantitative analysis of those assumptions. The accounting and finance group may be helpful in guiding this process, but the detail still remains the responsibility of everyone who is part of the planning process.

Finally, it is important to have the action plans generated from the bottom up: that is, to review in detail the smallest action, and drive upward to more significant issues. For example: when forecasting revenues, determine all of the action steps that lead to revenue recognition from the bottom up. Look at past referral activity, and project the expected referrals from each source on the basis of historical activity and current activity to generate additional referrals. This process drives for a connection between activity planned and results achieved.

Performance Measurements

Performance measurements that provide all participants information on how the enterprise is doing, as well as determining the accomplishments of individual members, are crucial to the success of the enterprise. Determining what to measure and how to measure it may be quite difficult. This difficulty arises when it is unclear what needs to be accomplished to fulfill the mission or when the goals are poorly defined. In either case, the difficulty reflects the larger problem of insufficient clarity to execute the mission.

The first step toward developing standards of performance is to determine what tasks need to be performed, and how those tasks are best organized and grouped by individual job descriptions. Once individual job descriptions are created and skills sets defined, the process of establishing standards of performance can begin. From the job description, clearly define the results that the person filling that role should accomplish. From this point, questions on the measurability of the intended results can be addressed. Some will be binary (either yes, it was met, or no, it was not), and some will be quantitative (for example, time line met a certain percentage of the time), able to be subjected to other statistical measures. In addition, providing mechanisms for how the data will be collected will be necessary.

Once performance measures have been established and tested for each function in the enterprise, a system of continuous improvement may be implemented. It is helpful to view the enterprise as a learning system in which all participants are in a continuous learning process and improvement occurs as people and systems evolve. This approach provides both insight into individual performance and a better understanding of systems that have been created to produce the intended results. Variation between goals and actual performance can be studied to determine improved methods, and trend lines can be developed to measure actual results produced in different time frames.

It is important to focus on producing the intended results, not just meeting preexisting standards that may or may not be relevant to producing the results currently required. Preestablished standards, rather than continuous improvement techniques, can drive individuals to short-term decisions that meet goals but do not produce the intended longer-term result. It is very important to understand that the measurement system is just a tool and cannot be expected to replace management judgment.

Performance standards may be an effective and positive way of communicating the intended results the enterprise is committed to produce. If they are viewed as a negative "watchdog" mechanism, however, they may have serious negative side effects. Management of the enterprise must provide complete communication about the standards and how they will be used to advance the mission of the enterprise. Participants of the enterprise need to see the larger picture to understand how performance standards can be useful to the enterprise and to the individual participants. Performance that does not measure up to the standard may offer an opportunity for the individual to learn and grow in his or her job. Continued poor performance, however, cannot be tolerated since it would send a clear message to the rest of the organization that nonstandard performance will be acceptable.

These are fine lines and only skilled and experienced managers can make these judgments accurately and consistently.

No text on operating performance would be complete without a discussion of cash-flow planning. While this function is generally provided by the accounting and finance department, all key participants to the planning process should be aware of the factors that affect cash flow. If cash flow variables are not considered an integral part of the planning process, a vital perspective will be missed that may substantially affect key assumptions. All participants in the enterprise generate cash and expend cash resources. It is very important that these individuals understand the impact of their actions and decisions on cash.

Audit of the Enterprise

The importance of iteration during the planning and implementing of a design for the total enterprise has been mentioned several times. The audit process that is intended to determine the feasibility of the organizational design to accomplish the founding vision and objectives acts to close the loop of the plan, thereby creating a circular design. The results produced by the enterprise should be reviewed periodically, usually on a quarterly or semiannual basis, depending on the maturity of the enterprise. This review should provide the process for asking and answering the following questions:

- Has the organization achieved the expected operating results?
- If so, were the accomplishments achieved as a consequence of the planning and implementation, or were there fortuitous circumstances that acted favorably on the enterprise? If no fortuitous circumstances are identified, does this suggest that goals were set too conservatively? If not, does this suggest that the overall strategic plan presents greater opportunity than originally planned?
- If the organization has not achieved the plan, what were the underlying factors that prevented achievement of the goals? Were there fortuitous circumstances that acted unfavorably on the enterprise? Were there breakdowns in the execution of a standard process or specific action plans? If so, what was the cause of the breakdown and how can it be prevented in the future? Perhaps these breakdowns will create a positive learning experience for the future. If less than favorable results were achieved, and no significant breakdowns are identified, results

suggest unrealistic goals were set during the planning process. If less than favorable results were achieved, and no significant breakdowns are identified, does this suggest a problem with the strategic plan? If so, how can we identify the area requiring further examination?

- What can we learn from the results, either favorable or unfavorable?
- How, given the actual history and current trends, can the enterprise alter the plan to produce greater accomplishment?
- Considering the results achieved, what seems to be the greatest challenge for the enterprise?
- Considering the results achieved, what seems to be the greatest opportunity for the enterprise?

The greatest challenge to having an effective audit process is the willingness of all participants to confront the issues realistically and constructively. If the audit process becomes an agonizing "blame game," the richness of the process will be destroyed, and the organization will slowly, but inevitably, begin wearing blinders that will result in plans and behaviors that are not consistent with the needs of the enterprise or the customers.

CONCLUSION

In conclusion, the design of an enterprise is a highly creative process that requires considerable discipline to gather and analyze data on which to build a useful plan to accomplish the vision of the enterprise. This responsibility is not for the faint of heart. Insufficient data on which to build a solid plan, uncertainty about the future in a rapidly changing health care environment, difficulties in producing a shared vision for the enterprise, and finally, the law of unintended results all conspire to frustrate the planners and managers of the enterprise. Because of these and other challenges in guiding the enterprise, successful accomplishment of the mission and the fulfillment of the vision become especially rich experiences for the participants of the enterprise and those they choose to serve. These rewards are even more significant when the enterprise has chosen to achieve specific outcomes that enable severely injured and/or ill people to return to happy and productive lives.

Case Example

To clarify some of the points discussed in the strategic planning section, a hypothetical case is now presented. Necessarily, the example given is an oversimplification, but it should serve to illustrate some of the major points discussed. While it is beyond the scope of this chapter to deal in detail with operational aspects of the plan, it is very important to stress that an exceptional strategic plan may fail if aspects of the plan are not completely revealed in a detailed operating plan. As indicated in the body of the text, the planning process is iterative and the reasonableness of a strategic plan can only be judged from a rigorously developed operational plan. Until the operational objectives that support the strategic plan are detailed in action plans, work flows, and pro formas, the plan cannot be rendered viable.

Background

The American Rehabilitation Institute (ARI), located in a large midwestern city, has provided inpatient and outpatient rehabilitation services to residents of the city and the surrounding area for over 40 years. The hospital is a stand-alone unit and historically received referrals from surrounding acute hospitals.

ARI is a nonprofit institution governed by a board of trustees. During most of the hospital's history, revenues exceeded expenses sufficiently to fulfill the institute's working capital needs. The facility and equipment were partially funded by donations, with the balance being funded out of the institute's revenues. However, since 1985 annual surpluses deteriorated and during the past 2 years the institute required operating funds to be financed out of previous reserves.

In response to the deteriorating financial condition, the board of trustees asked the CEO to form a task force to develop a new strategy for maintaining the institute's financial viability.

The Environment

When management evaluated the institution's current economic environment the following facts were noted:
- Admissions reached a peak in 1984 and had been gradually declining until 1993, when the decline accelerated.
- Since 1993, there had been two staff downsizings.

- The length of stay for inpatient services had been steadily declining.
- During the past 2 years the hospital had been approached by managed care companies who were aggressively pursuing rate reductions and per diems. Per diems combined with the shorter length of stay occasionally caused the cost of services to exceed the payment received.
- Recently other hospitals had entered into subcapitation agreements that would pay the hospital a fixed amount based on a formula calculated for a certain population. These payments then are made monthly based on the determined population. However, usage could vary considerably, making it very difficult to match unit cost to units of service.

The CEO decided to have full representation on the task force and to balance the efforts with clinical, financial, and marketing participation. After several meetings the task force decided to take three data gathering steps.

1. Review original founding documents to determine the purpose and mission of the institute.
2. Interview all permanent employees.
3. Conduct outside market research primarily focused on payers and referring institutions.

After several months of hard work the task force reduced the data collected down to the following statements:

- ARI was founded to provide specialty services for patients from the city and surrounding area who, through injury or disease, had physical and cognitive disabilities.
- The goal of the institute was to restore the physical and cognitive functioning of severely injured patients to the highest possible level consistent with available resources.
- When ARI was founded, most of the costs were covered by the patient, the patient's insurance carrier, or contributions from the city and its residents.
- Currently, most of the costs were being covered by the patient's insurance carrier or the state and federal government. Contributions on a per capita basis had steadily declined and were contributing very little to the institute.
- The clinical staff was very concerned about the pressures placed on the treating teams for reduced services, lower cost, and shorter lengths of stay.

- External case managers were very aggressive and frequently were perceived by the clinical staff as interfering with appropriate medical care.
- There was considerable rivalry between the inpatient and outpatient clinical staffs.
- The clinical staff believed that marketing was overly aggressive in promising outcomes and setting per diems.
- The marketing department believed that the clinical staff was "not living in the present" and needed to understand what was happening with managed care.
- Capacity in the marketplace had expanded greatly over the last decade. Many hospitals who previously referred patients to ARI had opened "specialty programs" that included beds dedicated to rehabilitation. Stand-alone outpatient clinics that competed for the same patient dollar had been created. Additionally several years ago a large chain located a full continuum of care for general rehabilitation services in one of the city suburbs. This had a substantial impact on patient admissions from that large suburban population.
- Several large employers had signed with a midwestern health maintenance organization (HMO) to provide services on a capitated basis. The task force had studied the benefits offered by the HMO and had concluded that rehabilitation benefits were more restrictive than the area's normal indemnity plans.

On the basis of these conclusions, the task force provided the CEO with a list of options.

- Completely redefine the institute's mission.
- Develop another major downsizing plan.
- Merge or be acquired by a fully integrated medical services enterprise.

The board of trustees ruled out merger or another downsizing. On the basis of the available information the CEO was instructed by the board to produce a plan for redefining the institute's basic mission and market position.

The CEO carefully reviewed the founding objectives. Were these objectives still valid given the excess capacity in the market? After all, when the institute was founded specialty rehabilitation services were not widely understood or available. In order to answer this question the CEO and the task force studied their data. The following conclusions were generated:

- The available capacity for general rehabilitation services far exceeded the market demand. However, as the population aged, the demand for services would increase. Additionally, other competitors might be weaker than ARI and withdraw from the market during the next 2 to 5 years.
- While it was true that supply exceeded demand, there was still a need for an organization with expertise in interdisciplinary rehabilitation for severe cases. However, focus would have to be on value for a particular patient population.
- The marketing research indicated that the institution's reputation among providers and payers for high-quality outcomes for serious cases was above that of the competition.
- On the basis of these data, the CEO concluded that there was still a need for a continuum of outcome-focused rehabilitation for injured and diseased members of the community that could best be met by the expertise of ARI. Hence, the founding objectives remained intact.

Where Are We?

The data assembled by the task force were used to present the overall picture for the institute. Clearly, a new vision and definition would be required to make ARI a viable competitor. On the basis of these data the task force concluded that ARI must decide to restrict its services to a subset of the market where measurably superior clinical outcomes could be achieved at optimal costs. Since many competitors could serve the market at large, the institute would focus on private pay primarily with workers' compensation carriers, reinsurers, HMOs, and certain large employers who would agree to carve out their accident and health benefits for illnesses and injuries that required major rehabilitation. ARI would attract these payers and their insured populations on the basis of risk-shared pricing and, in some cases, capitated pricing. Pro formas were developed that reflected revenue exceeding total cost within 3 years.

These projections were based on the following conclusions:
- Patient admissions would decrease as the result of moving to serving only the severely injured patients. However, this would be completely offset by offering carriers outcome-focused rehabilitation services under a risk-sharing pricing mechanism that would create an accountable partnership. Hence patient admissions were expected to grow.

- Revenue per admission would actually grow as the result of serving the more severe cases and offering a full continuum of services.
- Cost per unit of service would gradually decline as the result of implementing a continuous quality improvement program. Compensation of staff would be linked to performance and outcome accomplishment.
- Overhead would increase for 2 years while implementing new programs but would then decline as a percentage of revenue based on creating a flatter organizational model and decreasing marketing costs through a risk-sharing partnership model.

Definition

ARI will provide a full continuum of rehabilitation services for severely diseased or injured patients. These services will be provided to patients who are insured by carriers who have an ability to integrate outcome data with risk-shared pricing mechanisms and will work in partnership with ARI directing most or all of their patients to the institute. The catchment area will be the greater metro market.

This definition restricts the type of patients served and will target a certain type of payers who will work with the institute as a partner on a comprehensive basis.

Mission Statement

ARI will be the leading provider of outcome-focused rehabilitation services for serious injuries and illnesses in its marketplace. The institute will have satisfaction ratings above 95 percent from patients, families, and payers. Planned clinical outcomes will be achieved 98 percent of the time and per unit cost will be at or below standard 98 percent of the time. Revenue will exceed all costs within 3 years and reserves will increase by 5 percent of annual revenues each year after break-even is achieved.

ARI Vision

ARI will be a nationally recognized leader of outcome-based rehabilitation services. Carriers and providers who carry risk for patient populations will consider the quality of the outcomes achieved by the institution to be superior and recognize the value based on resources used as well as outcomes achieved. The institute will be seen as a role model that will allow ARI to recruit the best available clinical talent as well as being a national leader for developing critical paths of care.

Strategy

- Develop a proprietary outcome-based score card for the local market based on widely used national standards.
- Develop pricing mechanisms that relate performance to price.
- Be accountable for results, not process.
- Develop partnership arrangements with major carriers and employers to provide care for all of their patients.
- Develop a public relations strategy focused on the metro market for payers and patients.
- Concentrate treatment plans on the needs of the patient, rather than milieu or preconceived modalities of care. Plans should ask the question, What does this patient need to reach the highest functional performance possible and how can this be done at optimal cost? Turf issues will be set aside.
- Implement a process to collect data on the five most important cost drivers. Then implement a continuous quality improvement program to reduce the per unit cost associated with the five factors.
- Recruit leading edge clinicians who are committed to ARI's vision.
- Develop compensation systems based on team performance. With this system relate outcome to resources used.

In terms of these conclusions a detailed operational plan could be constructed to include specific action plans, the design of the organization, job descriptions, standards of performance, work flows, and detailed financial pro formas. Finally, the detailed operational plan could be compared to the strategic plan to ensure that a viable plan that is internally consistent has been constructed.

Chapter 9

Leadership

Pat Kitchell Landrum, MA, CCC, and Richard D. Hansen, MS, MSW

Objectives

- To distinguish leadership in being, language, and action.
- To provide an opportunity for readers to recognize leadership in themselves and in others.
- To present the relevance of leadership in the development and implementation of outcome-oriented rehabilitation.
- To demonstrate that when leadership is present, people are more productive and experience significant meaning and satisfaction.

INTRODUCTION

All of us can remember people we have met who have made a difference in our lives—a teacher, a supervisor at work, a colleague. We can recall stories about something that individual said or did that profoundly affected us. Moments with those individuals sometimes feel like a gift. Developing this chapter has been such an experience. Before we sat down to write, we reviewed some of the volumes of literature on the subject of leadership. To bring our reading to life, especially in the field of rehabilitation, we interviewed a number of individuals throughout the United States, identified as leaders by their peers in and outside the field of rehabilitation. In those conversations we began to distinguish just what leadership is. Our intent in this chapter is to give the reader a chance to recognize leadership in yourself and in others and to distinguish leadership in being, language, and action. Furthermore, our hope is that you will apply these distinctions in the development of a working rehabilitation system for the future well-being of American communities.

In this chapter we will assert that leadership is a crucial business distinction for the development and implementation of outcome-oriented rehabilitation. To change our industry from the traditional provider-driven process, an orientation that focuses on our activities in the treatment environment will call for leadership. Leadership will be required to change to a consumer-driven outcome-oriented rehabilitation process where we work from a projected result back into coordinated action. Leadership will be required to challenge our assumptions about who we are, what we do, why we treat, how we work together, and how we measure our process and outcome. Leadership is one of the building blocks that make an industry paradigm shift possible.

In the pages that follow we will invite you to reflect on where you see leadership to be present in your work and community context. What do you see happening in the people, actions, and outcomes when leadership is present and when it is absent? How does leadership occur differently in different contexts? When are you a leader? How can you develop leadership in your workplace?

As you read we hope you will see that people can actualize their leadership potential and operate as leaders in their workplace and community. They can come to distinguish the environmental conditions, behaviors, and accomplishments that occur when leadership is present. We hope you see that when the key principles of leadership are distinguished, potential leaders can choose to lead others to produce unprecedented results. We also hope to reveal that when leadership is present, people have more fun at work, have more energy for their lives, and maintain their well-being as a model for the patients they serve.

THE INQUIRY

We interviewed 22 individuals whose rehabilitation- or health care–related business experience ranged from 20 to 35 years. Most of the people we interviewed are nationally recognized leaders in more than one venue, such as business and professional organizations, and were referred to us by several independent sources. Our group of men and women included presidents, chief operating officers, and medical directors of hospitals and free-standing rehabilitation agencies; the chief executive officers of two national health care accreditation agencies; an executive vice president of one of the nation's largest health insurance companies; and a physician for one of the nation's largest health maintenance organizations. We interviewed entrepreneurs who serve on the board of several private health care corporations, venture capital leaders, as well as case managers, rehabilitation program directors, nurse managers, administrators, and clinical service leaders. We spent from 1 to 2 hours with each participant. In our interviews, we began by asking for a definition of leadership and its characteristics. We inquired about the differences between leaders and managers. We heard many stories about managers who had evolved into leaders, about leaders who had been influential, and how potential had been recognized and mentored. Our questions then moved into three areas:

1. What happens when leadership is missing?
2. How does leadership drive out fear?
3. How does leadership facilitate change?

This inquiry led to lengthy discussions about the changes affecting health care today, the vision that some leaders have for rehabilitation services in the future, and ideas about how to recognize and develop leadership.

We talked with both men and women who described their lives, the roles they have assumed, and their accomplishments. They shared their dreams about the future of rehabilitation as well as what happened to them personally and professionally as they broke through barrier after barrier to accomplish unprecedented results. We listened to these men and women recount stories about leaders who had influenced them in their lives. We heard these same people praise others they considered to be the future leaders of their organizations, and we listened with fascination as they put forth their visions of the future.

In this chapter we will share what we have learned. We will introduce you to some of the people we interviewed, and, like us, you may find yourself saying, "I would like to work with you; I want to share your vision."

WHAT IS LEADERSHIP?

In our interviews we recognized there was not a single definition for leadership. No two people we asked used exactly the same words to describe leadership. Often they listed characteristics that together painted a picture of their image of leadership. In those descriptions, however, common themes emerged that were very consistent with the literature in business leadership. In this section of the chapter, we will attempt to capture these characteristics and principles of leadership.

Among the people interviewed, there was general agreement that good leadership involves having a vision of a future, a sense of values, the ability to communicate effectively, and a capacity to understand the big picture. Leaders readily anticipate what is going to happen. They prepare themselves and their followers for it. Leaders have a sense of civility in the way they approach the people with whom they work. They are courageous; they take risks because they trust their beliefs and their vision for a different future. Leaders have a "service ethic." They have a deep belief that they must act in service to others. We heard that a leader is not unlike someone who conducts an orchestra, someone who has the ability to harness talent and channel it in one direction. "Leaders translate where we are headed and tell us why." Leaders "hold up a mirror in front of those they are leading." Another person stated it this way: "Leadership is really about how you ask questions and how you solve problems." "Leadership is an evolving process. It does not simply settle in a person, but dynamically grows in an individual or group."

One of the women we interviewed said, "A leader is a person or group of persons creating a vision of where a program is going." That comment opened up our inquiry about leadership being embodied in a group of persons. We wondered, how does a group or team develop as a "leader"? Is that group perceived as more effective because it is perceived as embodying leadership?

Another woman described many of her accomplishments over the past few years. She spoke of creating a new spirit within the organization and teaching people in the organization to grow with each new challenge. She recounted success after success throughout the organization and concluded, "I am very proud of what they have done." She assuredly believed she was not alone as the leader, and although she did not say it, it appeared that there was a group of people leading that organization who acted as one. This woman was one of many individuals who spoke of a spiritual sense, an inner force, that emanates from leaders.

We recognized in our interviews that leaders express themselves in distinct ways. They speak with authority but usually not as authoritarians. They readily share stories about themselves, including stories that describe times of vulnerability. As the president of a large rehabilitation complex put it, "I really screw up at times." When we queried one person about how she knows she has made mistakes, she stated, "When I get aggravated over the smallest things, I know I need to step back before I make the next move."

Finally, we observed through our interviews that results happen when leaders are leading. Outcomes are achieved and experienced as accomplishments. People report feeling energized and satisfied. Leadership is clearly present in a high-velocity results-oriented work environment.

In summary, the salient characteristics of leadership as they occur in people, conversation, and organizations are

- Vision
- Communication
- Integrity
- Ownership and commitment
- Trust and ability to take risks
- Humor and perspective
- Orchestration
- Service ethic

Leadership need not occur only at the top levels of an organization or team. It need not occur on a formal level. It may be expressed from any level in the organization to impact action and results.

As we continue to inquire into what leadership is, it may serve us to consider the possibility that leadership is not a product or set of personal attributes as much as it is a set of distinctions. These distinctions empower an individual, group, or organization to achieve specific results.

EIGHT DISTINGUISHING CHARACTERISTICS OF LEADERSHIP

Vision

Leaders in American health care describe vision as
- the ability to see a future worth attaining;
- the capacity to hold a vision in the face of no consensus;
- the willingness to take a stand for a future that others do not yet see;

- the talent to abstract a meaning, a focus, a purpose from the chaos at hand;
- the ability to focus the attention and action of many on one identified goal.

When leadership is present, the leader and the followers envision a future possibility that would otherwise be concealed, or unrecognized, as the goal. A leader may bring this vision to a group or create a safe environment for the group to invent a future. High-technology "skunk works" and off-site strategic planning retreats are examples of how a leader brings a group together to invent a vision. The characteristic of vision reveals that in a leadership rich environment, new futures become possible and are spoken and brought forth into action.

The leaders we interviewed all spoke to the role of vision in leadership. Some described their visioning work as letting their mind wander in the shower, following the play of their children, reading "everything" and relating it to the problems of the hospital and community, or listening to the patient and family for what is needed in the rehabilitation plan. Many of them spoke to the importance of being with and listening to the customers and noncustomers of the product or service as a key to vision and visioning. Peter Senge, in *The Fifth Discipline,* identifies shared vision as "one of the five disciplines of a learning organization."[1] Great leaders throughout history are remembered for their articulation of a vision: the Reverend Martin Luther King, Jr.; Thomas Jefferson; Madame Curie; Susan B. Anthony.

To move an enterprise, a team, a patient, or a family calls for vision, a way to share the vision, and a possibility of achieving that vision that matters to each participant in the venture. Outcome-oriented rehabilitation is visionary in that you have to set your sights on an outcome that is in the future. You then go through a process of *reverse engineering* that links where you are today with your vision of the future.

Communication

Health care leaders described communication as
- the give and take of information,
- the core skill of leadership,
- the way we make things happen,
- the ability to be with staff and allow them to be "real,"

- the willingness to listen to everyone, in all segments of the organization,
- the ability to make a vision clear enough for followers to follow,
- a capacity that is crucial to internal and external customers,
- a structure for fulfilling the vision of the organization,
- a way to create and follow shared vision.

Communication in leadership includes speaking, listening, and written communication from the most formal business plan to how notes are sent on e:Mail. One leader said, "I request people to confront their issues head-on with me. I give them as much support and information as is needed. I absolutely give my people emotional support, too." One leader described an open 2-hour lunch the first Tuesday of every month. Employees from throughout the system are invited to come and bring issues to his attention. They can argue an initiative, suggest improvement, and share market information. About these meetings, he said, "I usually have 10 to 15 people attend. I've received some of my best business development leads from these sessions."

Another leader revealed that she tells her staff to call her anytime. "I educate people around me to dispel any fear, emotional reaction, or misinformation about key issues. I use formal meetings, regular circulars, monthly reports, and lots of informal communication to keep the key goals in the front of every employee's consciousness. I want them to know always that every little thing this hospital does is related to being of service to the community and to the people. This helps them set their personal priorities and make sure that their day is structured to be a *quality improvement* day." This hospital CEO has a box of cards in her desk that she hand writes and delivers to staff to acknowledge contributions. She stresses how important it is to be clear on the purpose and intended result of every initiative that the senior management communicates to the organization. She always includes staff from a number of departments and from many levels of the hierarchy in key meetings. "The textbooks on leadership and quality are right. The principles are straightforward; we just have to do what we say and say what we do."

In a leadership enriched environment communication is complete in both content and quality at all levels. Gossip is not tolerated. All are empowered to notice, stand for, and speak for honest, complete communication.

Integrity

Leaders in the health care industry define integrity as
- completeness,
- honesty,
- possession of the mission and core principles "in your bones" under all circumstances,
- core values that show leadership are balanced,
- ability to face the facts and own mistakes,
- tough-mindedness and pure-heartedness,
- compassion,
- forgiveness,
- giving of credit,
- grace.

The principle of integrity is one that many leaders and followers know to be at the heart of taking a venture through hard times. The leader is willing to take credit when credit is due, and also to take "the heat" when things go wrong. The leader is able to see and express the "perfection" of the organizational life cycle and guide the venture forward. One of the people we interviewed told us, "When people are afraid, I don't judge them, even subtly, as it hurts the process. If I judge people who are whining, complaining, or crying, instead of assuring them, it just won't work. You have to understand where it is coming from."

In a leadership enriched environment, the participants are aware that the work at hand is greater than the individual ego. Individuals do not need to be recognized or held up to awe. People are able to give and receive credit for accomplishment freely. There is a sense of power without a need for drama. In a leadership enriched environment it is safe to listen to, be with, and communicate the truth. The words of leadership must match the true intent. When a leader does not "walk the talk," an organization can actually feel the lack of integrity. False communication erodes effectiveness whether it comes from the top or from a piece of gossip in the "ranks."

Ownership and Commitment

Leaders characterize ownership and commitment as follows:
- Leaders are willing to stick to their vision even in the face of no consensus.

- Leaders are committed to the game, to winning, and to their people.
- Leaders generate a shared vision.
- Leaders generate commitment that reflects personal ownership.
- Leaders need courage.
- Leaders provide commitment that is like a beacon when you are surrounded by chaos.
- Leaders have a core commitment that is the underlying stability that allows change.

Leaders throughout history have shown their followers that all players involved can share something great if they are willing to contribute to bringing forth that something. Shared commitment occurs as a leadership principle in the completion of a project or in the formulation and delivery of each rehabilitation plan for patients served.

In our interviews, many leaders suggested that the energy, inspiration, and feeling of abundance associated with shared commitment are available at all times. One person said, "Something worth striving for is just beyond the everyday view. The job of the leader is to unveil and unleash that gold mine for access to all." Many leaders spoke of their ideals and their ability to guide people toward shared commitment as a drive, as a matter of luck, or as a gift. Many agreed that for them results happened around them as leaders because they were able to focus the attention of the stakeholders on a "something" to be committed to. They saw their job as being able to articulate that "something" clearly enough so that all stockholders could see and own it within them. Their vision was paired with an attitude or will to achieve through shared effort.

Leadership is expressed through a *stand* for working on a project until the team has reached the right answer, through a team commitment to doing whatever it takes to achieve the target outcomes, and through a commitment to the people in an enterprise. Leaders create a community around the work at hand. The community has shared ownership of the project, the process, and the results.

Trust

American leaders say the following about trust:
- Trust is a firm belief in another's reliability.
- Trust is confident expectation.

- Trust lets one allow without misgivings.
- Trust inspires trust.
- Trust that leaders inspire enables them to press the edges of the envelope out.
- Trust allows leaders to show others that it is safe to take risks.
- Trust gives the leader assurance that the team will hold the enterprise to its course.

Generating trust and making it safe to take risks allow a team to invent a new future for an organization. Shared risk and trust enable the team to begin to act. We usually think that trust is built over time. In our interviews, however, we understood that it may not be time based. Leaders ask for and then honor the trust that has been given them. When leadership is present in an individual or in a conversation, trust emerges. This trust allows all participants to extend their performance synergistically.

Building trust in a time of change and reorganization is perhaps one of the biggest challenges an organization will face. Many times the leaders themselves feel ambivalent about helping to bring in the new order. Yet they are able to see the bigger picture, the necessity for change, and to provide the positive support to institute it successfully. "Leaders create an environment of trust and stability for change to happen." Once that environment is present, leaders can express their vision for the future and the path they will chart to achieve it. In reflecting on the role of leadership during periods of change there was a realization that openness to new possibilities was a critical attribute. As the president of one organization put it, "Leadership is not being invested in the past, not being so certain of what 'should be.' "

Leadership that engenders trust fosters creativity and innovation. It creates an efficient and productive working environment in which staff do not have to watch what they are saying or be concerned that there are hidden agendas. The critical aspect of trust is that it must be assumed in the environment. Everyone should be trusted until demonstrated untrustworthy.

For example, the section chief of a spinal cord injury rehabilitation team with a national reputation for excellence saw that a subset of patients in his program did not require the standard protocol of care. He saw this in the face of no consensus from his peer group. He did, however, present a proposal to his team to try a new alternative. He put his reputation at stake and dedicated substantially more time to the management of the initial cases on the new service to assure the integrity of the plan and to confirm his hypotheses. This action generated a shared trust and willingness to take risks in both staff and patients.

Sense of Humor and Perspective

Proven leaders described humor and perspective as follows:
- Humor is a sense of proportion.
- You have to be willing to laugh at yourself.
- Humor is critical to taking risks.
- Laugh at it, laugh with them, laugh at yourself, keep your humor.
- We must look beyond the next week, quarter, and year to five years.
- Each challenge is a great challenge but not the end of the world.
- Look ahead; don't get too focused on the details of now.

Leaders have to maintain and generate a perspective on the current goals as well as on the new goals. The ability to have a sense of humor about all aspects of the enterprise while honoring it is one of the artful aspects of leadership. One leader we interviewed said, "When working with other people's fears this depth of understanding is critical. Once a leader understands what created the fear, he or she has the opportunity to turn that fear around, creating something totally different, so that everyone can move forward." Another told us, "When I get scared I do a lot of self-talk and ask myself, what is the worst thing that could happen? At work, we talk a lot about our failures to gain perspective and then deal with them."

For example, one director of quality for a multisite rehabilitation company told us about her executive development program. She asked her managers whether they were willing to have quality breakdowns be a gift and a lesson on more than one level. Her job included investigating patient and family complaints, incidents and accidents, and licensing preparation with the facilities. On the matter of perspective, she said she always reminded directors and managers to consider the plight of the trauma patient when the manager was losing perspective. "Imagine the possibility that it takes you 10 minutes to find shoes in the bottom of your closet. Then imagine that after 10 more minutes you still are not sure if the shoes match. Now, look at the data in your situation. Put it in perspective. The facts are always good news because you know where you stand." Leadership enriched environments allow the participants to see what happened as a learning opportunity.

Organization and Orchestration

Leaders we interviewed discussed organization and orchestration.

- The leader must see how to make things happen.
- Organization is the ability to have the action of the enterprise managed for result.
- Leaders must see how to balance and integrate change.
- Most good leaders know how to use a good manager.
- Organization of an enterprise is like being an orchestra conductor.
- Leaders can anticipate and prepare the organization for change.
- Many leaders are not managers but know how to identify and ensure management.

One person said, "Managers traditionally have been rewarded for acting in logical ways to accomplish the goals set by the organization. They rely on the leaders in their organizations to recognize the significance of that sensibility." Leaders may be supporting one level of project management while initiating a new way to accomplish the larger mission of the organization. A woman who manages a large physician practice said it another way: "I see where I need to take the doctors. I see what their resistance is now and what it will be later. My job is to be aware of the three-dimensional nature of leading from this administrative position. The elements of this juggling act include knowing who I am at all times, knowing and respecting my physicians, appreciating the scope of their work and their needs for recognition, knowing where I want to take them, and knowing how I can make their day go more smoothly today so that they will do it in a new way tomorrow."

This element of orchestration and integration is as relevant to ongoing operations as it is to innovation. The work of leadership is not focused only on innovation, change, and development. In a leadership enriched environment, the daily routines of maintenance can take on the meaning of excellence. Leadership enables a group of people to do the same things over and over again as a ritual with meaning as opposed to drudgery. When leadership is present, a balance between stability and growth can be maintained. Leadership draws attention to the value of coordination, flow, and completion.

Service

In our interviews, the service ethic was characterized as

- listening and responding to the real and perceived needs of others;

- looking inside oneself at all times for resource, energy, and inspiration;
- being ready to serve when the situation calls for it;
- creating a context for straight talk and truth;
- being open to new ways to serve others.

Leaders can make things happen by standing for them and maintaining a relationship to workers in a way that infuses action with meaning. Many of the leaders we interviewed spoke of their service ethic as a way of being with others. It is an attitude of being responsible for success while giving accountability for achievement to another that then enables the accountable person to become truly empowered.

The service ethic is exemplified by a middle manager in a large county hospital system surrounded by specialized proprietary businesses. She is recognized in the region and the industry as a leader, although she does not see or describe herself as such. This woman has been working "in the ranks" for 10 years and chooses to do so. She sees her job as keeping all therapy staff positions filled, keeping the union in partnership with the hospital for minimal grievances and work stops, and delivering "the best care" to hospital users. This leader at the operations management level is inspired on a daily basis by the opportunity to be of service to the community. Her leadership is demonstrated by successful union management relations, regional recognition of the facility for quality, and high staff satisfaction reports.

LEADERSHIP IN ACTION

"People tend to want things to stay the same, to do things the same way even when they're in the change business," was the comment of a physician leader of a large rehabilitation enterprise. "I'm the apostate," he said, "I get tired of doing the same thing and so I'm continually creating new ideas and acting on them. I gravitate to new challenges."

He didn't start out as a physician, but along the way in his career he thought medicine was a genuine challenge. Soon after finishing his residency he formed a group practice, but after building a successful practice, he needed a new challenge so he became the medical director of a short-term stay hospital.

Not one to be limited to services inside the hospital, he soon developed a number of outpatient services and even managed and owned a congregate living facility. Today his work carries him to a number of states and his influence is national in scope. How does he manage to keep expanding? He says simply, "Total quality management."

His leadership skills are focused on physicians. "Physicians have a personal value of quality, but do not always have a way of measuring it and today third-party payers want it measured. I work hard to get physician cooperation. I've found that having quality coordinators work side-by-side with physicians gives dual commitment to a project or process." When he speaks about quality this physician leader also emphasizes the importance of being cost-effective and delivering the right outcomes in order to secure and retain third-party contracts.

We further learned from this physician leader that physician involvement in quality goes beyond clinical quality. It includes quality in the way a patient experiences an office visit, a physician interacts during a telephone conversation, or he or she speaks at a staff meeting. "To be very practical," he said, "we're a for-profit entity and patients and families have many options. I want them to choose us."

As he explores new avenues of service in the rehabilitation community this leader told us he keeps challenging the existing paradigms of care. For instance, now that there is less of a need for general acute care beds in community hospitals, he sees an opportunity to turn some of those unused beds into rehabilitation beds. These same facilities have an existing outpatient base that might also benefit from a rehabilitation presence in the community. Working with existing hospital administrators and physician leaders at a number of hospitals, he has been able to introduce the local health care leadership to a variety of rehabilitation services in their own communities. He and his staff bring the expertise necessary to provide high-quality, cost-effective rehabilitation services closer to home.

We wondered after interviewing this physician leader what new ideas he might suggest the next time we talk with him. We are certain that whatever he creates in the future will bear his stamp of quality and innovation. This leader in action demonstrates all eight characteristics of leadership.

LEADERSHIP ASSESSMENT

How does one identify leadership, assess its development along a continuum, choose to grow it or appoint it? In our interviews we explored a number of aspects of leadership assessment. We looked at the traditional question of nurture or nature. We explored whether women and men lead differently and whether leadership appears in different ways depending on the context. We inquired about how to identify whether there is sufficient leadership available to transform an organization or an industry, and how leadership drives out fear, facilitates change, and fits with management. We asked what an organization looks like in the absence of leadership.

Almost all of the leaders we interviewed said that they could tell when leadership in the organization was lacking. "The fish starts to smell from the head." They saw that to move any enterprise forward requires leadership. They saw this as essential because in the absence of leadership "the ship stalls in the water." They agreed that particularly in the emerging health care market of today there is more need for leadership than in the past. Historically, health care was relatively stable. It was staffed by people who liked stability and could move forward deliberately according to a 5-year plan. Today, that is no longer sufficient.

We heard many stories of what happens in an organization when leadership is missing. Chaos takes over. "The wheels fall off." "The enterprise runs out of steam." "People begin to look out for themselves and get political." "In-fighting and pettiness take over." "Results just don't happen. People talk about things but do not make decisions or stick with their commitments." "People focus on everything except their goals." In the absence of leadership there is an increase of blame, fear, and resignation. Confidentiality is violated.

Well-recognized leaders agreed that almost anyone in an enterprise can *feel* when leadership is missing. It takes an insightful manager or a person with an understanding of the core competencies of leadership, however, quickly to *identify the missing element* as leadership.

The performance drift described occurs in the absence of leadership. It occurs when a position is left vacant for an extended period or eliminated without clear reallocation of accountability. It occurs when an individual is appointed to a leadership role but does not function as a leader. It occurs when a manager overcontrols and squashes leadership. It happens when a group of people are forced to "operate in a vacuum" or asked to change without access to contextual information. It often happens when responsibility and accountability are not aligned around results in a management matrix. It occurs when the responsible person has no accountability for changes. It occurs when management and union or employee and management goals are not aligned or expressed.

Teams, departments, divisions, and hospital systems lose their engine when leadership is absent.

Those we interviewed stressed that rehabilitation services require leadership. They agreed that in the absence of leadership, organizations do not meet their full potential, customers notice that something is missing, and workers for the enterprise are not fully self-expressed. In the absence of leadership rehabilitation providers could lose their role as decision makers and become victims of a faulty health care reimbursement paradigm. It behooves managers, line staff, and powerful leaders in rehabilitation to identify, cultivate, and promote leadership in their organizations because as we move into the next millennium, there is a lot at stake.

In our interviews we learned a lot about what leadership is not. We heard it said that visionary thinking in the absence of responsibility, ownership, and integration is not leadership. Forcing people to do something through the use of threats, punishment, bribery, or lies is not leadership. Efficient management without vision, communication, and commitment is not leadership. *Leadership* is not another word for the identified boss on a project. Heroics and dramatic performances are not leadership.

On the question of nurture or nature there was a wide disparity of responses. Most of the men interviewed believed that leaders were born. Women tended to answer the question by describing how they had moved through their organizations and how they had been nurtured and mentored by someone who had believed in them. Both men and women agreed that some people appear as natural leaders and that these naturals respond quickly to mentoring. One of the women we interviewed introduced the idea of creating new leaders by saying, "I've been seeding ideas. Some of these ideas are growing and leaders are emerging to take them to harvest." Men spoke of identifying and then challenging potential leaders. Most of the time they labeled these people as natural born leaders. The authors, consultants who are hired to identify and develop leadership, agreed that potential leaders are easily identified, that tools and distinctions of leadership can be taught, and individuals in key leadership roles can be coached to empower their full leadership potential in context. What follows are some tools for you to apply in identifying and growing leadership in your organization.

WHY DO YOU NEED LEADERSHIP?

As you seek to develop leadership in your enterprise, what is missing that leadership will nurture?

- To deliver on the basics of the business?
- To hold parts of the enterprise more closely to manage change?
- To support the business in tolerating pressures from the field and/or other parts of the organization?
- To deepen the quality of service to your customers?
- To design and implement a new process to produce results?
- To develop a new service line?

WHAT TYPE OF LEADERSHIP IS NEEDED?

Knowing what kind of leadership is needed will assist you in seeking out the right people for development or in focusing your own attention for personal growth.

- Situational leadership?
- Team leadership?
- Division, service line, or department leadership?
- Professional network leadership?
- Organizational or overall business leadership?

These different leadership needs may call for different levels, depths, and experiences in leadership. For example, a service line manager may seek to develop situational leadership in all staff. The manager would educate staff about leadership characteristics, build a leadership development element into staff supervision routines, and reward demonstrated situational leadership.

A rehabilitation unit director may seek increased team leadership in the case managers as more managed care contracts are implemented or in department heads as the facility experiences an overall decrease in staff. In this case, the rehabilitation director might recruit new managers, contract a consultant to implement with current staff, implement a formal plan, or send key managers off-site for leadership training.

The board of directors may seek overall enterprise leadership. The search committee would seek an individual with a proven track record in most, if not all, aspects of leadership.

LEADERSHIP POTENTIAL

Several key questions will guide you to leadership potential in individuals.
- Do these people see and articulate the big picture?
- Can the individuals communicate up, across, and down the organizational lines?
- Is their behavior consistent with their word: that is, do they walk their talk?
- Do they take risks but manage to stay "inbounds" with their initiative?
- Can they keep their eye on the goal while enrolling others at the case, situational, and/or project level?
- Can they tolerate failure and frustration without becoming angry or resigned?
- Can they keep their balance in a complex environment under pressure?
- Can they prioritize and produce results on time?
- Can they shift priorities without unnecessary resistance or resentment?
- Can they shape the behavior of others, and mobilize resources effectively?
- Do they act in service of others, the mission, and the goals of the venture?
- Do they demonstrate performance or potential in your specific targeted and technical areas?

After identifying whether an individual meets your basic screening criteria, you may wish to engage in a dialog to determine whether the individual is interested in pursuing leadership training, or engaging in a leadership development relationship in context. If *you* are interested in developing your own leadership, consider participating in a personal leadership development program. In either case, select a mentor and a coach who will work with you to establish goals, processes, and feedback sessions. Establish a time frame for development and clear results that will emerge from leadership development.

Identifying strengths, weaknesses, knowledge gaps, and opportunities for development is the next step in developing leadership. The Leadership Assessment Plan (Table 9–1) can be used to guide the assessment and development of the leadership student. This tool provides a vehicle for identifying strengths, weaknesses, action plan, time frame, and specific mentor or guide.

In Table 9–1 the Leadership Assessment Plan has been completed for a hypothetical new leader in training. Areas of focus and dialog are completed; areas that will not be a focus are left blank.

THE LEADERSHIP DEVELOPMENT PLAN

Having developed a view of strengths, weaknesses, areas to study, and environments where leadership can be expressed, evolving leaders should work with a coach to create a focused action plan to achieve specific benchmarks in time. This leadership development plan targets specific behaviors from the key leadership areas, actions to be taken, and measures for accomplishment. The leadership coach or mentor works directly with the leader in development, to look at the surface behaviors of leadership in action and to assure that the underlying principle is distinguished. The coach helps the developing leader to apply skills to a variety of settings. The mentor or coach is always identifying ways in which the principles of leadership are relevant to the activity at hand and to other situations as well.

Formal Leadership Training

There are a number of educational opportunities available to individuals interested in developing their leadership skills. Most universities and colleges offer some kind of program dedicated to personal and professional advancement. These programs acknowledge the growing need for strong leadership in a variety of areas, including health care.

Two programs with proven records are provided by the American College of Medical Practice Executives (ACMPE). One of the programs is held on 5 consecutive days and the other is usually held once a month for 12 months.

The 5-day program sponsored by ACMPE and the J. L. Kellogg Graduate School of Management at Northwestern University encourages the participation of teams of physicians and administrators who attend class together. They are encouraged to support the idea that leadership is often enhanced when team members understand each other's leadership style and, therefore, complement each other's strengths and weaknesses. In this program participants look at what determines an organization's corporate culture so that they can understand their own organization.

Table 9–1 Leadership Assessment Plan

New Service Line Manager
Time Frame: 6 Months

Target Area	Weakness/ Strength I II III IV V	Action Plan	Date Completed	Who Will Help
		Vision		
a. To be able to see and/or generate a vision.	Strength 5	Build on this strength by initiating a "break-through" project that will call for producing shared vision and powerful action.		Facility leader or professional peer.
b. To communicate vision for others to see.	Strength 3			
c. To hold that vision in the face of conflict or disagreement or no consensus.	Weakness 2	Present proposal to XX opponents; practice; prepare.		Immediate supervisor
d. To abstract a meaning, a focus, a purpose from the chaos at hand.	W 2	Learn to stand back, collect data, generate hypotheses.		Leadership coach
e. Other–Select one or more other characteristics.				
		Communication		
a. To be able to generate a context and purpose for accomplishment.	S 4	Use this skill to express vulnerability in weak-ness and solicit help.		Workplace peers; supervisor
b. To be able to facilitate dialog.	S			
c. To be able to facilitate conflict resolution.	W 2	Breakdown conflict to sub-parts. Resolve small conflicts before tackling big ones. Use dialog skills.		A colleague who is good at it.
d. To facilitate problem solving.	W	Observe.		Read case examples from "The Goal", a colleague who is good at it.
e. To translate key messages to different levels of the organization.	S			
f. Other–Select one or more other characteristics.				

continues

Table 9–1 continued

Target Area	Weakness/ Strength I II III IV V	Action Plan	Date Completed	Who Will Help
		Integrity		
a. To demonstrate the core values of the organization.	S 5			
b. To "walk the talk."	S 4			
c. To face the facts and own mistakes.	W 2	Own my mistakes. Identify these; share them with mentor.		Leadership mentor
d. To tolerate frustration.	W	Learn to read my frustration. Learn to develop a quick frustration & error barometer. Speak of these regularly with peers, supervisor & direct reports.		Leadership mentor or immediate supervisor.
e. To give credit.	W/S 3	Give credit for accomplishment to individual(s) in workplace at least once a day.		Develop a checklist.
f. Other–Select one or more other characteristics.				
		Ownership & Commitment		
a. To hold that vision in the face of conflict or disagreement or no consensus.	W 3	Post-vision statement. Know you won't always win the first time. Speak vision in all settings.		Immediate supervisor.
b. To generate commitment because of personal ownership.	S			
c. To demonstrate courage when the vision may be questioned.	W 2	Continually reflect on the vision when questions arise about it.		Take time alone; ask a colleague to help.
d. To represent stability so that change can happen.				
e. To stick with the vision until a project is completed.				
f. Other–Select one or more other characteristics.				

continues

Table 9–1 continued

Target Area	Weakness/ Strength I II III IV V	Action Plan	Date Completed	Who Will Help
Trust				
a. To be able to trust in oneself and in others.				
b. To be able to sustain an environment of trust.	S			
c. To be able to manage the creativity & innovation that results from an environment of trust.	S			
d. To show others that it is safe to take risks.	S/W	Learn to be more confident so you always create a safe environment.		Immediate supervisor; coach for soliciting feedback.
e. To reward those who return trust & generate it in others.	S			
Sense of Humor & Perspective				
a. To be willing to laugh at myself.	W 2	Separate personal and business; notice the value.		Closest friend at work.
b. To point out the humor in situations in order to create perspective.	S			
c. To recognize that humor is critical to taking risks.	S			
d. To recognize the big picture, especially when surrounded by details.	W	Learn to distinguish details from big picture; stick to the big picture.		Immediate supervisor.
e. To look ahead; to keep the future in mind.	S			

continues

Table 9–1 continued

Target Area	Weakness/ Strength I II III IV V	Action Plan	Date Completed	Who Will Help
		Organization & Orchestration		
a. To recognize the difference between organization & orchestration.	W	To read more about leaders & managers.		Ask the President of the organization for recommended reading.
b. To recognize the role of managers and to support them.	W	Same as (a).		
c. To know how to draw on the skills of different managers.	S			
d. To recognize that the organization exists to serve the mission and the vision.	S			
e. To anticipate & prepare for changes in the organization.	S			

Leadership styles may work well in one culture but not in another. Once you discover where you work best you can develop your leadership skills to their fullest. Role playing in these classes also offers the opportunity to test your style with a colleague as well as with leaders from other organizations who may be willing to point out characteristics that impede your ability to lead an organization. As a result, participants learn to emphasize their strong points, work on their weak points, and/or recognize that they need a fellow team member to complement behaviors they cannot change.

The Northwestern experience provides an opportunity for participants to review some of the basic skills needed to support leaders in the fast-changing world of health care. Courses in finance and business strategy, along with negotiating skills, offer role playing opportunities that sharpen a participant's ability to think and act quickly. Rounding out the week is an in-depth look at total quality management, concluding with a course examining the principles of effective change management. Participants leave this power-packed week with a renewed sense of their own leadership potential.

The 12-month program includes many of the same courses in the 5-day program. What differs are the length of each course and the time between courses. Most participants comment that the intervals between classes afford the opportunity to test theories taught during the previous month. Having a chance actually to introduce a new idea or style of practice in an organization helps to ensure that it will not be forgotten.

The 12 courses offered in the ACME Management Education and Development Series (MED Series) are similar to those in most business schools, with the practical applications directly related to the health care issues of today. For instance, 10 hours of strategic planning offer leaders the opportunity to think beyond their day-to-day paradigms, and to consider possibilities for the future. At the same time, courses in finance, accounting, and human resource development ground leaders in the practical knowledge needed to ensure an organization is moving in the right direction.

The MED Series faculty promote the philosophy that physician leaders and other health care professionals need a solid foundation in all aspects of health care management to build effective teams to manage the present and create the future.

The Make a Difference Group—an Example

In contrast to formal leadership education programs, many organizations implement in-house leadership programs and many consulting groups provide individual or small group leadership development products. One such program was implemented inside a moderate-sized multisite rehabilitation company through a partnership of the CEO, the vice president of clinical services, and a transformational management consultant.

The program was offered to a small group of employees throughout the organization, including business managers, clinical staff, sales and support personnel who had demonstrated leadership potential and a commitment to "make a difference." The program included two 3-day off-site intensive sessions, participant projects, and structured telephone calls over a 6-month period. During the off-site training sessions participants distinguished leadership, committed to bring leadership to their operation sites, and designed projects whose implementation would require a dramatic leap in leadership.

The program coordinators coached them in project completion and generalization of the leadership training into the facilities of the participants. As a result of implementation, the Make a Difference program produced unprecedented clinical service and business results for the company. Several participants moved to higher levels of responsibility and accomplishment.

CONCLUSION

Leadership is both a set of skills and a way of being with other people. The eight distinguishing characteristics of leadership presented in this chapter can be applied individually or with groups as a model for leadership assessment and development.

Our intent has been to show how leadership can be distinguished and applied to increase the effectiveness of rehabilitation practice at many levels. We hope that we have demonstrated that leadership is not a nebulous art but can be grounded scientifically, just like rehabilitation practice.

The way to implement what we have presented in this chapter is to
- apply the distinctions,
- choose to put yourself at risk,
- be your word and say that is what you are doing,

- use information and data responsibly to guide your action and decisions,
- look for the truth in the matter and follow it,
- learn to apply dialog to go to the root cause of issues,
- achieve alignment on initiatives instead of simple consensus,
- work from the whole with the whole organization,
- empower people to make the leaps necessary to get to new ground,
- ask for help, ask for feedback, and take it seriously.

No matter how a leader chooses to develop his or her leadership skills, whether it be in a mentoring relationship, at a local college, through a national educational program, or through a professional association, it is important to challenge oneself continually. A true leader is always learning, always open to new insight and to new ventures. It is possible for every individual to be more of a leader than he or she is now. There is nothing to lose. Set a functional outcome target and go for it.

We wish to acknowledge the many individuals who contributed to this chapter. Although we do not have room to mention them all, we wish to specifically thank Sister Lynn Casey, Dr. Edmond Charette, Mary Cunningham, Craig Davenport, Dale Eazel, Don Galvin, Dr. Bruce Gans, Judith Lazar, Dr. John Melvin, Sue Murphy, Dr. Anna Pomfret, Barbara Scheffel, Errick Woosley, and Mary Kay Moore.

REFERENCE

1. Senge PM. *The Fifth Discipline*. New York: Doubleday; 1990.

SUGGESTED READINGS

Agyris C. Teaching smart people how to learn. *Harvard Bus Rev.* 1991;3:99–109.
Bennis W. The pivotal force. *Enterprise*. 1985;9:9–11.
Bowen HK. Regaining the lead in manufacturing. *Harvard Bus Rev.* 1994;5:108–140.
Epstein C. Ways men and women lead. *Harvard Bus Rev.* 1991;1:150–160.
Huey J. The new post heroic leadership. *Fortune*. February 21, 1994:42–50.
Rinpoche S. *The Tibetan Book of Living and Dying*. San Francisco: Harper; 1993.
Stewart T. How to lead a revolution. *Fortune*. November 28, 1994:48–61.
Wheatley M. *Leadership and the New Science*. San Francisco: Berrett-Koehler; 1992.

Chapter 10

Transformational Management

Joseph D. Friedman, MA, and Pat Kitchell Landrum, MA, CCC

Objectives

- To introduce a theoretical framework for the organization of limited resources to produce excellent outcomes and a high degree of customer satisfaction.
- To present six principles of transformational management with associated tools and techniques for application of these principles in rehabilitation.
- To describe additional practical tools for efficient management within the discipline of transformational management.

Introduction

Health care is changing. Payers are demanding cost reduction without quality reduction. Rehabilitation managers are being asked to produce better outcomes with fewer resources. As the percentage of health care dollars being spent inside managed care contracts increases, more and more providers are being asked to promise specific outcomes for set fees.

More than ever before the role of rehabilitation managers is critical to the organization's success and even survival. This chapter is an introduction to managing in a way that is uniquely suited to the rehabilitation environment. Our intention is to present a theoretical framework for assisting the organization of limited resources to produce excellent outcomes, and to offer a few practical suggestions for adapting this method to the reader's unique management challenges.

Transformational management works best in those situations where a team, department, or organization is committed to accomplishing a critical result for which the pathway to accomplishment is not yet clear. One might call such an accomplishment a *breakthrough*. Breakthroughs are needed where thinking and techniques that have been effective in the past are no longer adequate.

Rehabilitation service providers in the 1990s are faced with the need for breakthroughs in many areas associated with health care reform. The successful past history of managing rehabilitation planning, service delivery, and business does not address the gap created by the dramatic changes in the industry that are occurring today. Merely doing more of what has been already tried will be insufficient. Doing the same thing better will also fall short of what is needed. Even doing something different in the same context will fall short of a breakthrough. It is possible to produce incremental improvement in outcomes by changing the behavior inside an existing context or paradigm, but *breakthroughs* result from a fundamental shift in context. Transformational management is a methodology for intentionally causing and sustaining breakthrough outcomes.

Managers are by nature results-driven and often impatient with abstractions and theory. The authors request the reader's patience with the more abstract portions in this chapter. Likewise, we acknowledge that in some instances we are using common words in a specialized way. We are, in fact, presenting a jargon. We have attempted to limit the use of jargon to the minimum we consider essential to give our readers a clear sense of how this management technology truly differs from more familiar approaches.

In this chapter we present six principles of transformational management and a section on management tools and techniques consistent with the principles. For each principle, we will give a brief introduction, an example of application, skills to build, and practices that will help in applying the principle.

We have seen the application of transformational management, as presented in the pages that follow, produce outstanding results in many instances, in many different venues. Our hope is that this introduction will contribute to readers' ongoing quest to produce better outcomes for their clients and their organization, while increasing their own and their staff's level of satisfaction. This chapter is not a comprehensive presentation of transformational management. We refer you to resources listed for further exposure to the discipline and opportunities for deeper learning.

FIRST PRINCIPLE: TO CAUSE A BREAKTHROUGH IN RESULTS, SHIFT THE CONTEXT FOR ACTION

Intentionally managing context is one of the distinguishing character-istics of transformational management. By *context*, we mean the frame of reference for an action. If managers can impact the context in which their staff are operating, they can cause radical shifts in behavior. Such radical shifts are the source of breakthroughs.

In the sense we are using the word, "context" and "being" are virtually synonymous. By "being" we mean a set of linguistic constructs that make up the sum total of all our frames of reference. Things for which we have no context quite literally do not exist for us. Who we *are* pre-cedes our experience. It is not information or knowledge that generates behavior; it is being. We are, we perceive, we act.

The question of *being* is usually overlooked because it is not normally deemed the province of management. Managers earn their keep by having those they manage produce results that would not happen without the inter-vention of management. What is predictable doesn't call for much manage-ment. If management's job is to cause nonpredictable actions or breakthroughs, then it behooves managers to discover those concepts, tech-niques, and practices that would allow them to access the domain of *being*.

What makes *being* accessible on an everyday basis is to distinguish it as a network of conversations through which an individual interacts with the world. In this regard the *being* part of *human being* is composed of both stated commitments such as "I stand for open, honest communica-tion" and unspoken, unconsciously held commitments such as "No mat-ter how hard I try, I lose," or "If I always appear cheerful, I'll be OK." In an organizational context the aggregate of these conversations make up the *organizational being*, or culture: "It's not what you know; it's who you know. We can have either high-quality care or profits, not both. Nobody gets acknowledged around here. They kill the messenger in this shop," and so on.

In both individuals and organizations, the power of *being* is evident. At a small rehabilitation hospital in the Midwest, we encountered a case manager, Sue Ellen, who was behaving consistently with an unidentified silent conversation that went something like "My boss never listens to me." (All of the names and locations mentioned in this chapter have been changed to support confidentiality of clients served.) More than simply thinking this thought, she was *being* and dramatizing the proposition "It doesn't work to speak forthrightly around here." Sue Ellen did not present new ideas in the unit management meetings. She would rather manipulate her innovations into action during case conferences and informal conversations with staff over lunch and in the hallways. Sue Ellen was operating inside an unconscious context that limited her freedom of action. The way she was being, her context for herself at work, was slowing program development and causing confusion for the team.

The first step in causing a breakthrough with Sue Ellen was to introduce the concept of "mental models." The idea of mental models is fundamental to transformational management. This concept is based on the assertion that what we experience is not absolute reality — it is reality as it occurs for us, and that what occurs for us is a function of our mental models. When mental models are not distinguished as models, people behave as if their interpretation is reality, in fact, people behave as if they aren't interpreting but merely responding to real situations that dictate a given response. When individuals grasp the importance of mental models in determining behavior, there is often a sigh of relief because the possibility of freedom that then arises. When Sue Ellen was able to distinguish the thought "My manager never listens to me" as an interpretation rather than something fixed and "true", she became free to create another interpretation of the manager's behavior, such as "My manager really is interested, but first I have to get her attention," and then to behave consistently with that model.

After Sue Ellen shifted the context for her relationship with her director, her behavior began to change naturally. She began to introduce her innovative ideas using unit management protocol. In an e:Mail sent to the director, Sue Ellen requested time in unit management to introduce a new idea. Presenting her new idea as a written proposal to unit management, she included the purpose, the intended result, the proposed innovation, and a strategy for a trial in her team. In a meeting with her director, Sue Ellen explained that she was eager to be creative and try out new ideas but was fearful her ideas would be rejected without trial. She then asked the director to support her attempts at introducing innovation.

The outcome of confronting that silent conversation that limited the relationship with her manager was a breakthrough. This breakthrough yielded an increase in clinical case conference efficiency, better clinical results, and an improved relationship between the manager and her director and set the stage for further high-velocity change in the department.

Getting one's arms around context and one's hands on being does not assure automatic success; one still must execute. It will, however, give the manager a critical, competitive edge.

Skills to Build

- Discerning context
- Separating interpretation from fact

Practices

When problems arise, ask oneself about the invisible framework or context in which this action is occurring: What are the unseen limits on behavior in this situation? What are the habitual ways of being shaping behavior in this situation?

SECOND PRINCIPLE: THE PRESENT IS CAUSED BY THE FUTURE

This concept of action in the present being caused or correlated with the future is counterintuitive. Our ordinary thought process is linear, as is our relationship with time. We live inside a mental model that goes something like, *what happened in the past is causing our actions today.* This model is pervasive and not often questioned. If this deterministic model is correct, there is nothing we can do other than react to the present; since the past cannot be changed, the die is already cast.

It is certainly true that we live *as if* we are coming from the past into the present and on into the future. Once an event happens and we respond to it successfully, a mental model begins to be formed about how to handle that situation *or anything that resembles it.* What is guiding our present behavior are our past interpretations and conclusions about how to succeed. The future we have in this mode of thought is a future filled with the past. Breakthroughs occur when we are able to create a future that takes the past into account but is not limited by it.

Transformational management rests on the premise that it is, in fact, possible to create commitments that are not reactions to the past that will drive our current behavior. By commitment we mean *an explicit statement of serious intent regarding the **future***. Commitment is not considered to be a feeling, but rather what one has said in the past about how one will be in the future.

Commitments can exist at the levels of both awareness and nonawareness. Commitments about which we are unaware have the power to undermine more consciously determined commitments. A commitment that is, in fact, *freely chosen* and not a reaction to something that happened previously gives a new paradigm or context for present action. It gives a new *possibility* for action.

The normal understanding is that a *possibility* is something that we predict has a weak chance of occurring, such as "I don't think so, but it's a possibility." It may also refer to one of a range of options, such as "Which possibility will you select?" In the context of transformational management *possibility* carries a special meaning. A possibility is an *invention,* a newly created statement about what could be. The actions taken in the past that gave the organization the results it currently has were the expression of some possibility. If we want a breakthrough, it will be necessary to create a new possibility, not simply change behavior inside the one we already have. Possibility and paradigm, in that respect, are similar concepts.

A possibility exists first only in language. A possibility is a nonmaterial creation that then allows for actions that ultimately are expressed as tangible results. That which exists is an expression of that which was possible. Transformational managers have their ears tuned to the language of possibility.

To invent possibilities is not to fantasize. One cannot declare the department highly profitable when it's in the red, and then expect the budget actualities to change magically. One can, however, declare the *possibility* of being profitable and begin to operate out of that possibility, rather than merely react to being unprofitable. The difference is subtle but profound. Inventing and acting on a possibility does not ignore the past; it involves a clear understanding of current realities that is complete and clear. Present actions are unencumbered by myths about how the past, present, and future are linked.

For example, at a midwestern hospital and rehabilitation center, the inpatient and outpatient rehabilitation programs had separate managers and distinct staff. Patients discharged from inpatient services were admitted, evaluated, and treated by the hospital outpatient staff as if they'd come from a different facility. The outpatient program was not included in the initial rehabilitation planning process when the patient was admitted to the inpatient unit of the hospital. When transferred to outpatient, the outpatient staff developed new goals and objectives for the patient from an individual discipline perspective in occupational, speech, and physical therapy. These conditions were an expression of an established organizational culture. That was just the way it was and had been for 20 years.

Bob, the new vice president of operations, trained in the discipline of transformational management, saw that inside the current context for operations there was no possibility for simultaneously meeting the hospital's right-sizing requirements and maintaining standards of care. Bob was committed to something beyond what had been attainable at this hospital for 20 years.

Bob met with the managers of inpatient and outpatient care as well as the department heads for all therapy disciplines. He acknowledged the contributions that each manager had made in the past and stated the hospital's commitment to their continued employment and growth. He led the team in rigorously identifying what was currently so about the unit's operations. He then created an environment where it was safe to speculate and launch half-baked ideas, without the ideas being shot down immediately as impractical. He coached the team to listen actively for the positive benefit in each new idea and to build consciously on the previous suggestion. He made sure the team refrained from "voting" and continuously kept expanding the limit of what they all could imagine. He paid careful attention to the degree of enthusiasm and inspiration in the group, a sure sign that possibility is being created.

After each participant shared his or her vision for the hospital, the VP of operations engaged his managers in a dialog in which together they invented a *new possibility*. Each patient admitted would have access to a seamless continuum of care that transcended departments and divisions. They then went on to invent a new delivery system. Once this new possibility was fully created and documented, Bob and the management team held additional meetings. They examined practicality, cost versus benefit, and other considerations before getting into action on the possibility they had designed.

Ultimately the management team created a new model of care that had neither discipline departments nor inpatient and outpatient divisions. Six management positions were eliminated. Case managers and treatment teams were empowered to follow patients across in- and outpatient stays within diagnostic programs. The number of inpatient beds was reduced. The diagnostic programs implemented an integrated rehabilitation plan and documentation system that was carried through all phases of patient access to the system. The hospital established a strategic partnership with a subacute program and local home care company to provide the additional elements of the hospital continuum of care.

The actions taken inside the new possibility allowed the hospital to reduce management costs, consolidate staffing pools, simplify billing and documentation, and reduce the cost of service by 12 percent over the 6-month implementation period. Regional and in-house referrals increased. The program exceeded all previous revenue and profit targets while retaining its standards of care.

Our experience with Andrea is another example of this principle. Andrea was clinical director of a free-standing program that had seen a reduction in referrals from hospitals. She also held accountability for negotiating funding. In the course of a meeting with an internal consultant skilled in transformational management, she realized that in her fearful reaction to the downturn in referrals, she was habitually and without conscious awareness being "the righteously indignant expert." Andrea recognized this stance was negatively impacting her program's sales, funding, referral management, and actual service delivery. It was at this moment she became free to stand for another way of being with the situation — to create a commitment about the future that would shift her actions in the next moment. The new commitment she made was "to be a guide and mapmaker for new ways of cost-effective treatment."

Once Andrea noticed how she had been "being," she was able to choose a more effective stance toward the situation to shift her commitments. When she felt herself falling back into her automatic righteous indignation, she now had a choice of being some other way. The future she had created for herself opened up a new way of dealing with the current challenging circumstances.

This shift opened a broad spectrum of new actions. Andrea no longer reacted to naive customers with disdain. She took the opportunity of their requests for program rationale to educate them about the possibilities presented by the program service. She no longer insisted on being the only person in the program to complete funding discussions with payers, allowing her case managers and assessor to provide information in support of funding decisions. She encouraged her case managers to create "blended" programs that were outside the "pure" program model, including variations of service consistent with those requested by the referral source. She empowered her field assessor not only to complete the patient assessment, but to contact the patient's insurer for funding approval at the referring hospital site within a simple set of program parameters. In her funding proposals, Andrea altered the amount and presentation format of patient data sent to the payer, reducing detail and program-specific jargon.

The results of her creating a new future, a new possibility for herself, included a dramatic leap in program admissions, a shorter referral to admission cycle time, an increase of diagnoses admitted to the program, and fewer requests by the payer for additional documentation before program authorization. In addition, the program increased funding types and length of program authorization. Andrea's behavior produced the results. "Upstream" of her behavior was a shift in *being* and conscious commitment — a shift in the kind of future she was committed to having.

Skills to Build

- Identify the interpretations, conclusions, and firmly held beliefs that shape the perception of the present situation, giving rise to present action.
- Support staff in designing new commitments for the future.
- Learn to speak in a way that inspires a sense of what could be possible without invalidating the past or present.
- Generate enthusiasm and inspiration.

Practices

- Spend time sorting out fact from interpretation. Discover where the past has colored the present.

• Set up specific times to invent new possibilities.
• Train oneself and staff on how to let conversations develop without immediately evaluating the feasibility of what is.

THIRD PRINCIPLE: TO CREATE A NEW FUTURE, ONE MUST FIRST RELEASE THE GRIP OF THE PAST

A powerful relationship to the past occurs when one has moved beyond reacting to it to accepting it. In the jargon of transformational management, this is *to be complete* with the past. Being complete shifts our relationship to the past. It enables us to create a new future.

The concept of *completion* addresses our attitudes, thoughts, and feelings about the past. Regardless of what we do or say, the past is, in fact, finished. It is possible, however, for something to be finished and not *complete* for us. When we are not complete with an interaction, situation, or event, there is something about the past that remains as a concern or even an "upset" for us. Whenever anything in the present reminds us of that about which we are incomplete, we reexperience the upset to some degree. As a result, rather than being clear-headed in the present, we are dealing with a present situation through the filter of a past upset.

When we *are complete*, the past no longer encumbers us. We can clearly see that past event free of emotional reaction to it. In this sense *completion* is a state of being. In that sense, it is possible to be complete with things that are not finished. Being complete does not imply that you agree with something in the past that you did not like. It simply means that you are no longer reacting to it.

The transformational manager realizes that being incomplete is one of the greatest impediments to creative solutions for today's management challenges. Think of your current workplace. Where is forward movement blocked? Is that block related to an incomplete past? If you were unencumbered by your feelings, attitudes, and opinions, might you see and pursue a novel solution to the block?

To *be complete* requires adopting a perspective of personal responsibility for the matter under consideration. To *be complete* means giving up the point of view that anyone or anything did it to you. This concept can be difficult to embrace in an organization where there is cultural agreement about being victimized and in which blaming is common-place. It is, however, an extremely useful idea to grasp. When an individual or group owns what has occurred then releases blame, shame, or guilt and declares that he or she is *complete with the past,* the next natural thing to do is create a new *possibility* and move forward. The following case example illustrates this principle.

The rehabilitation program in "F" Medical Center had a developmental history laden with false starts, management errors, and repeated turnover in program management. There were associated problems in service delivery. The hospital culture included normative beliefs such as "The hospital doesn't hire on the basis of competence; they shift the burden to avoid union trouble" and "You can't get fired here" and, "They don't care about quality." This organizational culture was demonstrated in both language and action on the unit. After 1 year of operation, the unit staff had elaborated this conversation to include such beliefs as "This place is not committed to excellence," "They won't change anything here," and "They don't know anything about rehab."

After 3 months in her position, the new program director saw that the culture she had inherited was unresponsive to traditional management intervention and would thwart achievement of second-year goals, possibly "burning her out." She contracted a transformational management consultant to lead a 3-month intervention, designed to give the department the basis for creating a positive future that was not predictable, given its past. The first phase in this breakthrough project was to *complete the past.*

The staff participated in an inservice introducing the distinctions of *possibility and completion.* A series of sessions to *complete the past* were held with each shift of staff, including managers from affiliated hospital departments, crossing all disciplines. In these meetings a safe environment was provided for the staff to communicate resentments, disappointments, withheld communications, failed expectations, and thwarted intentions. At the conclusion of these sessions all staff members were able either to release the past or to make a plan of action that, when finished, would allow them to be released. Before they could declare the past complete some staff felt that there were people outside the department with whom the staff members felt they needed to communicate. Upon a critical mass of completion, the program director invited the team to join her in a new commitment, that this unit would be a regional leader in providing state of the art rehabilitation.

The unit management team was restructured on the basis of each individual's spoken commitment to patient care, customer service, profitability, and results. The program director implemented a clear operations plan including weekly priorities, progress reports, and visual displays for the unit. After 1 month, staff performance in all target areas had improved dramatically.

Customer satisfaction reports and new referrals increased. To sustain accomplishment and continue to build this new culture committed to outcome-oriented rehabilitation, the program director integrated a process of continuous completion into her management and staff meetings. Each week staff were encouraged to acknowledge accomplishments of the past week, as well as communicate anything else that had not yet been communicated, in order to keep the department "present" with itself.

In summary, the impact of completing the past and building an ongoing culture of completion allows a team, unit, or enterprise to achieve durable outcomes and unpredictable accomplishments. Traditional management skills do not access and release blocks to resourcefulness that lie in the background of any group of human interactive processes. When the transformational manager augments proven skills as a manager with the distinction of *completing the past,* work can be completed more efficiently, blocks to movement can be addressed powerfully, and people can have a lot more fun at work.

Skills to Build

- Learn to identify when individuals or teams are encumbered in present action by attitudes, opinions, and assessments about the past.
- Learn to identify when an individual, group, or team needs a session to complete the past formally.
- Guide meetings or individual conversations for completion.
- Create a safe environment for communication of charged issues.

Practices

- Schedule regular sessions where the accomplishments and failed intentions of the past unit of time are acknowledged.

- Be complete in each interaction.
- Assure that the meeting is "clear" of an incomplete past before embarking on new work at hand.
- Take the time to go the extra mile for complete communication.

FOURTH PRINCIPLE: THE NATURE OF THE ATTENTION WE GIVE A SITUATION DETERMINES HOW IT WILL OCCUR FOR US AND HOW WE WILL RESPOND TO IT

We base our responses to the world on what we hear, see, feel, or sense. We do not act on what is there in reality, but what is there *for us*. It is now a truism that no one attends the same meeting. Like the blind men describing the elephant, we each encounter reality through our personal filters of perception. A critical part of the discipline of transformational management is identifying these filters or archetypes in the design of human attention. Once one has identified the automatic ways of attending to the world prevalent in a person, team, or organization, it is possible to learn to shift those ways of attending purposively.

An easy way to access this principle is through the window of communication, that is, through focusing on the subtleties of speaking and listening. The art of management requires the ability to take a familiar concept such as listening and imbue it with a new meaning. The transformational manager does this by helping others learn more about the design of their attention through the silent aspect of communication called *listening*.

What is heard is a function of the kind of attention an individual gives to what is being said. In this context, *listening* is not something you do, but rather a way of being. *Listening*, in this sense, is beyond the physiological phenomena of hearing. It refers to how one is predisposed to interact with what is present in the environment. It precedes perception and *allows* for perception. Our actions are based on our perceptions. Listening impacts on results inasmuch as the listening or mental model one applies to a situation determines what is perceived. We are generally oblivious to the listening we bring to a conversation and the listening that our colleagues bring. All our attention is usually on the speaking that is going on.

In order to design our own attention and the attention of others consciously, a few background assertions must be integrated into a group's working context. The transformational manager acts to create a high-performance culture by sharing the following assertions:

1. *Listening* is a generative, not passive, phenomenon. The *listening* one gives another determines the power and effectiveness of communication within that relationship.

For example, on a recent transatlantic trip, one of the authors was seated near the wing by a window. As the plane prepared for takeoff the flight attendants spoke about the plane's safety features, a talk we had heard dozens of times before. The attention given was consistent with a mental model that could be summarized as "I already know this." Although there was nothing wrong with our hearing, and the flight attendants were speaking quite clearly, none of what they were saying made any impact.

About 45 minutes later I heard a loud bang. I looked out the window to see a hole almost 3 feet wide in the leading edge of the wing right near my window. The metal was peeling back in the rush of wind even as I watched.

Two minutes later the flight attendant began to make an announcement about our flight. I heard every word as if it were engraved on my soul: same ears, same noise level, different quality of attention. In this case, the circumstances dramatically changed and so did the listening. A transformational manager learns to shift listening intentionally, not only when the circumstances dictate a powerful, appreciative attention.

2. There is a design to the way human beings *listen* when they are not aware of their attention.

More and more the job of management is to manage relationships. To accomplish this, a new level of self-awareness is required. To observe how we are being in the moment is a high art and an important skill for a manager to master. A critical element of the discipline of transformational management is *the knowledge of the design of attention or listening*. A manager who is clear on the design can work appropriately with that design to impact performance.

In this model, it is important to observe that in relation to what is happening right now, people are either present or not present to it. They are either with what is, or, "checked out." People often laugh in recognition when reminded of how often they and others carry on conversations with people *we know,* are "checked out," and then expect what they have said to have registered.

Simply penetrating the "politeness" that causes staff members to fail to mention to their colleagues that they are not present with them while communicating can cause real improvements in the efficiency of communication. The senior management team of a neurologic specialty provider learned this simple distinction, and began each meeting with a "clearing" to ensure that all members were present. If someone's attention drifted during a communication, it would not be uncommon for her to acknowledge that and request a repeat. When team members "called" each other on being checked out, it was invariably done in good humor and was well received. The results were improved communication, camaraderie, and meeting effectiveness.

Unless we consciously choose to pay attention in a different way, we will automatically take all input through a binary filter designed to promote our individual survival and control. At its simplest expression, the filter is simply a "right/wrong" sort. Just as a green filter on a light source will shade all objects in green, regardless of the content, whatever is attended through such a filter must be either right or wrong.

The predisposition to process new information through the binary system of right/wrong takes place at a precognitive level. It is more like a reaction to what is happening than a choice about how one will be. Before individuals begin to think, what is thinkable has already been determined by the filter. Without thinking about it, we *are* that things are right or wrong: it's *who we are being.* These habitual ways of being shape what is possible in a conversation without ever being noticed. In an organizational context this automatic way of being, left unchecked, squelches creativity, innovation, and full communication.

Other examples of automatic or reactive filters are derivative of right/wrong, such as good/bad and agree/disagree. Others are less closely related but serve the same function, that of unilateral control by listener. These include either/or listening such as "This change will be good either for management or for labor." Another common automatic listening is "What's the point?" This *listening* implies "I'm very busy. If I give you my attention, it is costing me, so you'd best get to the bottom line in a hurry so I can get back to more important things." What is important to note about these automatic listening filters is that no conscious energy is required to operate inside their parameters.

The transformational manager is interested in this phenomenon because these automatic ways of being with communication limit what is possible. If someone is presenting a new idea and the only way others have of *being* with that idea is through automatic or *reactive listening*, that new idea may be discredited well before it has had a chance to be explored. Worse yet, an organizational culture may grow up where people will not even speak up unless they are certain that what they say will be considered "right," or unless they have maneuvered within the politics of the organization so that their speaking is *listened* to respectfully.

It is possible to become aware of our reactive filters and design *proactive listening*. To *listen* proactively is to design one's attention so that it registers something different than what the automatic filters would allow. For example, one could intentionally interrupt the drift to reaction when a staff member approaches with a communication about her insights about what is wrong with the referral to admission process, and *listen for what is possible that I had never thought of before*. In this instance, the listener is *pulling* for possibility. The fundamental concept to grasp here is that we are not merely passive receptors of data. The kind of attention we give a situation determines what will register for us. We are constantly, and quite literally, creating the reality in which we operate by the way we are attending to the raw data presented to us. Listen for possibility and there it is. The Pygmalion effect is notorious. When the teacher begins "listening for" the student's excellence, the student tends to show up as excellent.

The list of proactive *listening* filters is limited only by one's imagination. One could shift the automatic tendency to listen for win/lose to listening for win/win, or from either/or to both/and. A particularly powerful proactive filter is *listening for commitment*. When D., a senior occupational therapist, went to the director's office, she was often carrying a complaint with which the director felt compelled either to agree or disagree. After coaching from a transformational management consultant, the director realized that she could interrupt her automatic agree/disagree listening and listen for D.'s deep commitment. It is important to note that underlying this technique is the assertion that our world is not separate from us, and that the way D. is occurring for the director has everything to do with the listening the director is giving her. When the director changed her listening for D., her behavior changed and the director's experience was different. The director began to discover the opportunity in D.'s challenging input and was able to create some innovative solutions to long-standing problems.

Another example of applied proactive listening is *win/win listening*. In a Midwestern hospital, the heads of physical therapy (PT) and recreation therapy (RT) often saw their goals as being in conflict. The head of PT automatically listened to the RT director through the mental model of win/lose. When she was introduced to these principles, she shifted her listening to win/win. Inside this shift in listening, the RT director's proposal to lengthen the community outing time no longer looked as if PT would lose treatment time with patients. The PT director could set her listening for win/win and see the possibility to cotreat with RT while out in the community.

The single most important proactive listening to adopt in order to facilitate communication, and build and develop trust in a highly charged environment, is a *listening for how it is for another*. When one adopts this way of being, one becomes committed to hold in abeyance the normal agreeing and disagreeing, and opt instead proactively to let into our own reality how the world is occurring for the other person. This way of being requires true vulnerability, a letting down of our defensive routines and letting in, really letting in, the way it is for someone else. This way of being is similar to empathy, but distinct. Really listening for how it is for someone else does not mean you even understand it: you have simply duplicated the experience in yours. Listening for how it is for another is a real challenge when what is being communicated is something negative about us, with which we don't agree.

When people experience that another has really heard the way it is for them, they feel known, appreciated, and respected. The communication is then complete. There may be further action that is required, but the speaker will not need to repeat the same communication over and over again, often dramatizing it in ways beyond words. A new level of trust and relationship has been established.

In today's managed care environment each of us must move rapidly and apply shorthand techniques in many areas of concern to meet our business, service, and clinical targets cost-effectively. Sometimes in our effort to move quickly, we hurt one another's feelings or offend one another. Because we are trying to work efficiently and maintain a smooth facade of relationship, we may be inclined to minimize any negative feelings that accrue during the course of our work lives. Unfortunately, nega-

tive feelings do not disappear of their own accord. The subtle buildup of
these hurts and upsets will ultimately cause a dramatic slowing of forward movement in the organization. Learning the skill of proactive *listening for how it is for the other* can release the buildup of incomplete,
internal conversations; keep the work space clear; and help create an
environment of active, mutual support.

The following vignette makes clear that the application of this skill
does not require a great deal of time or facilitation:

> Steve and Ann, managers in a California rehabilitation hospital,
> worked together on many shared proposals. They were both
> familiar with transformational management methods. On one
> particularly important proposal, Steve presented it in a way that
> did not include Ann's perspective. She was hurt and offended.
> She thought it meant that he did not want to work with her on the
> project, and that he had excluded her deliberately. Her interpreta-
> tion of that incident began to interfere with the daily work, which
> called for close coordination and partnership between them.
>
> Ann realized she needed to be in full communication with Steve
> in order that their working relationship be returned to a function
> level. Their conversations went something like this:
>
> "You know, on the call last week something happened for me
> and I want you to hear how it was for me. I don't need you to
> agree or apologize. I just want you to hear it. OK?"
> "Okay, how long will this take?"
>
> "Just a minute. Can we do it now?"
>
> "Okay."
>
> "When you changed your action plan in that presentation with
> Don, it seemed to me that you excluded my perspective and I
> felt like you wanted this project for yourself. I invested a lot in
> this and felt hurt by your actions."
>
> "Oh, I see that you felt hurt. Do you want more information or
> do you want me just to get that you feel hurt?"

"Just listen. I felt hurt that you excluded my work. I feel like you don't really want my contribution. So why work; get it?"

"Wow, I get how you feel and appreciate you letting me know. I didn't realize that you felt that way. Do you want an apology or an explanation?"

"Thanks for listening. I would like the data. I want to know what is next on the project and how you want to work together. Now that we have cleared this up, I can get refocused on work."

In this brief exchange Ann communicated how it was for her. She was able to get the facts straight about what actually happened and what the next project step was. In a relatively short time span, given their familiarity with the concepts outlined in this chapter, they were able to restore their relationship to full power. Their manager's investment in educating her staff in the method of transformational management produced an excellent return in strengthened staff relationships and an expanded capacity for accomplishing organizational objectives.

Skills to Build

- Teach yourself and others to observe the design of attention.
- Distinguish filters of attention and their impact on relationships and communication effectiveness.
- Learn to hold off your automatic reactions and intentionally duplicate another's communication.
- Learn to tell when another has actually heard deeply what has been said.

Practices

- Share your mental model and/or listening for a person or situation.
- Acknowledge when you or another is checked out.
- Establish eye contact while speaking.
- Limit facial cues while listening silently.
- Ask to be heard through the filter of *getting how it is for another.*

• Share with another that you are going to listen to him or her proactively through the filter of *getting how it is for another.*

FIFTH PRINCIPLE: COMMITMENTS CLEARLY EXPRESSED SUPPORT SUSTAINED HIGH PERFORMANCE

Transformational management focuses individual and group attention on *commitments* in order to accelerate the velocity of accomplishment. A *commitment* is a statement about behavior that will be. Just as attending to the unspoken, silent component of communication, attention, or listening pays handsome dividends, so too does learning and mastering a simple set of distinctions in speaking. Speaking in this context refers to all forms of communication, including memos and e:Mail as well as verbal expressions.

There is so much speaking going on in contemporary culture that people are complaining of information overload. As with any commodity, when it seems there is an endless supply, talk begins to appear cheap. In the discipline of transformational management, practitioners attempt to rehabilitate the power and value of our speaking. As with listening, the first step in this process is to examine the design of "normal" speaking in your organization. As the manager teaches each design element to his or her staff, an environment gradually builds for more powerful, effective, and efficient conversations, moving the work forward with more velocity and less effort.

The first design element is that most speaking is couched in language appropriate to describe what has already happened, *even when speaking about the future.*

When something happens in individuals' environment, they have a reaction to that change. They express that reaction. The verbal expression is linked to what has already occurred, what lies in the past. It may be the expression of an opinion, an emotion, or an attitude about what happened — all past-based. Likewise, there may be a careful analysis of the past quarter's admissions and length of stay statistics, and then a hypothesis will be offered about the next quarter's length of stay figures: sound management practice, of course, but all past-based speaking. To cause a breakthrough in outcomes may require more precise matching of tool to job, to using language suited to causing new futures as distinct from language suited to describing past occurrences.

The second design element of speaking to consider is that people's opinions and interpretations are often presented as the truth. Nothing kills dialog in a team faster than the failure to distinguish opinion as opinion. A place to begin the transformation of work-related conversations is the distinction of opinion/assertion. An assertion is a statement about the world for which you are prepared to give evidence. Assertions are testable.

The third design element of speaking involves making a distinction between language that describes something or represents something and language that generates something. For example the word *chair* represents chair and it obviously refers to the object that is described by that word. However, when someone says "I promise," the word *promise* does not describe anything, nor does it represent a promise; it is the act of promising itself.

The distinction "language that performs work" enables managers and staff to take the next leap in learning to speak a language that expresses, rather than hides commitment. For example, when someone asks another to produce a written report, saying, "I'd really like to get that report sometime," to which the other replies, "No problem" or "I'll look into it," what result has actually been produced in that interaction? The request is ambiguous. The commitment inside the request is ambiguous. Much of the wasted effort in organizations can be traced to the failure to speak and listen from a position of clear commitment.

The fourth design element in a matrix of committed speaking is to distinguish language that creates a future. A prediction is a statement about the future based on an analysis of the past. A prediction is a "talking about" something. A good manager needs to be able to predict. For breakthrough outcomes skill in prediction alone is insufficient. The manager needs to learn and practice the art of power *declaration*.

A declaration is distinct from a prediction or a statement of probability in that it does not describe a future that already exists nor talk about one that might. A declaration *creates* a *possible* future. That possible future then exists in language, not yet in physical reality.

The possible future or context for action that exists is critical to staff morale. A story is told of a man wandering the streets of Rome. He comes upon a stone mason chipping a block of marble. He asks the man, "What are you doing?" The mason replies, somewhat testily, "Chipping marble, obviously." A few strides beyond, the wanderer encounters another mason engaged in the identical activity. He asks the same question and this man answers, "I'm building a cathedral." Which person experienced more satisfaction at day's end?

A *declaration* can take many forms. The most common are as follows: "I declare _____." "I stand for the possibility _____." There is real power in having teams or individuals express *declarations* out loud. This activity becomes powerful when people are clear on the distinction of *declaration* and can see that they are, in fact, inventing something *in the act of speaking itself.* A declaration is the first step in bringing something new into existence. To declare something obviously does not make it true; it does, however, make it possible.

For example, the program director and team at "F" Medical Center declared a possible future for the team. Then, as the team did the day-to-day work of the department, they were doing it inside that possible future.

The director shared the distinction *declaration* with the group and invited the staff to declare the team's future with her. In a staff meeting, each person stood and declared his or her commitment to be on the team. They were inventing who they would be in the matter of this team. The staff declarations included "You can count on me to do whatever it takes to meet our goals." "I am on the team. I may have to be flexible with my hours because my kids have doctor appointments this month, but I will cover my schedule in advance." "I stand for helping this unit break all hospital records for customer satisfaction. You can count me in!"

As each person spoke his or her stand, it created a context of shared commitment. In their speaking the staff created their future as a team. The program director and medical director began to use declarations to set the tone or context of all their meetings. The use of declarations deepened the unit's understanding of committed speaking and their background of commitment to a shared future.

Declarations, once understood, can become the heart of outcome-oriented rehabilitation. The team, in explicit declaration of commitments, is dedicating attention and resource to the target outcome before initiating the rehabilitation process. Without the future-oriented language act of declarations, treatment teams and rehabilitation enterprises are at risk, with no clear links among process, outcome, and price.

The fifth element of committed speaking is communication for action. The simplest and most common elements of conversations for action are *promises and requests.* A *promise* is a spoken commitment to another for a result in time. A *request* is the speech act for soliciting a complete promise.

A *promise* is different from a *declaration.* A *declaration* is an invention of possibility. A promise is the statement of a specific action that will occur by a specific time, under specific conditions. A promise is grounded in commitment but is more focused and concrete than a declaration. It is the tool for moving a declaration into action.

The classic form for *promising* is "I promise *the specific result* by *some specific point in time.*" Promises can only exist in an environment where individuals place a high value on the integrity of their speaking. They are committed to the commitments they make; they are not "windbags." It does not mean they keep all their commitments. It means they take their commitments seriously. When they see they are unable to meet their commitments, they communicate about that to the appropriate people responsibly.

Transformational management requires going beyond the notion that it is good to keep promises and bad to fail to fulfill them. That morality actually inhibits people from promising anything they are not sure they can deliver, making the promise a weak tool. A transformational manager consciously creates a milieu where the integrity of communication is highly valued. Of course, there may be consequences for repeatedly making and failing to keep promises. That performance issue would need to be dealt with as such.

Requests are the corollary of promises. A request is the speech act for soliciting a complete promise. The classic form of requesting is "I request X by time Y." The responses available are "I accept," "I decline," "I counteroffer X," or "I promise to respond to that request by time X." Every one of these responses moves the work forward powerfully, including the refusals. One roadblock to the effectiveness of this tool is that it is unsafe to say no in many organizations. Part of the work of implementing a program of transformational management is to create an environment in which there is room for authentic declining. A true no is much more useful than a false or grudging yes, which only later reveals itself in the form of late or incomplete work.

In the event a manager genuinely cannot accept a no to a request, he or she is, in fact, making a demand. For example, within a case conference the case manager may say, "In order for Ms. Smith to continue her stay on the unit, I must submit the progress data and plan summary today at 3:00. I have to have the data and plan on my desk by noon. I know this demand may cause some other work to be delayed, but it is the priority right now." Demands are legitimate tools of management. They are more powerful when they are clearly articulated as such.

When all the elements of committed speaking are present in an organization, the quality of communication takes off and the velocity of action increases dramatically. Meetings cease to be awash in everyone's opinions and reaction only, and the conversations that occur actually move work forward. New possibilities are declared and a sense of inspiration and freshness can grow. As staff become comfortable with making promises and requests, there is an inevitable increase in the velocity of accomplishment. Nirvana, however, has not been reached. There are still problems, stuck places, and interruptions in the flow of work toward targeted outcomes.

Skills to Build

- Create a safe environment for people to express clear commitments.
- Discern opinions from assertions.
- Manage conversations to produce powerful declarations and complete, precise promises and requests.

Practices

- Use the precise forms of committed speaking until they become second nature — no short cuts.
- Track promises and requests made in each meeting as a measure of meeting productivity.
- Indicate respect for people's declarations, promises, and requests by listening to them intently, writing them down accurately, and having them typed up and shared appropriately.

SIXTH PRINCIPLE: SUCCESSFUL OUTCOMES ARE BASED ON WELL-HANDLED BREAKDOWNS

Winston Churchill said, "Success is going from failure to failure with no loss in velocity." The sixth principle of transformational management rests on the assertion that created, planned action is superior to reaction or inaction. The time when organizations are least likely to be in creative action are when serious problems arise. In this section we will present an approach to managing those "moments of truth," which occur every time the flow of action toward its end is interrupted. Another name for those moments of truth is "breakdowns."

As one moves forward toward a goal there are inevitable interruptions in the flow of accomplishment. The most common response to such interruptions is a negative reaction. The magnitude of the negative reaction is directly proportional to the size of the commitment to achieve the result that has just been interrupted, and that provides a clue to dealing with problems powerfully.

Transformational managers learn to be adept at handling problems in a way that minimizes the "down time" spent in reaction, and how to empower themselves and those they manage to use these situations as opportunities for learning and innovation. The velocity of accomplishment and the rate of innovation will increase as managers learn the skill of shifting from frustrated reaction to creative action, with ease and effectiveness.

The first point to master in building this skill is to explore the point of view that no situation is inherently a problem. The value we give the situation comes purely from our commitment. If I have no commitment to being in communication with anyone and my phone stops working, I do not get upset. If I am expecting a critical call on which my next 6 months' income depends and my phone malfunctions, I am frantic! When we take this point of view, the inevitable problems or breakdowns that arise become opportunities to review and renew our commitments, rather than occasions for invalidation and blame.

The second element in learning to deal creatively with breakdowns is to realize that *everyone*, no matter how enlightened, initially becomes upset when something interrupts his or her movement toward a goal. As soon as the interruption or breakdown occurs, there is an immediate reaction similar to "Oh no, not again!" Then there is the universal tendency to react as if something is wrong. Depending on our nature, individuals will speak and behave as if something is wrong with the other person(s) involved, with themselves, or with the whole system in which the problem has occurred. The automatic response to problems is that something is wrong, blame should be assigned, and the problem should be fixed immediately.

Transformational managers, when faced with such a circumstance, must both realize and be responsible for these automatic reactions and be committed to leading their staff beyond them quickly. Their goals will be to train the staff in shifting from the domain of assessment ("ain't it awful") or an assessment of the assessment ("ain't it awful that it's awful") to the domain of commitment and action.

Reviewing for a moment, we see that once a commitment to action has been made, there will be breakdowns in the flow toward accomplishment. In the face of such problems there is a tendency to blame, moan, and complain. John Whiteside[1] in his book on transformational management, *The Phoenix Agenda*, calls this juncture in the process of accomplishment a "moment of truth — a decision point that makes clear that the way we have been operating is no longer adequate." He postulates that facing such moments of truth "may be the *only* means of achieving exceptional results."

The third element in breakdown management at the "moment of truth" is consciously and intentionally to call a halt in the reaction to the problem, and declare a commitment to resolve it. The departmental management team discovers that they have seriously underbilled for their services during the last quarter. After the normal upset subsides, the team leader calls a meeting to address the situation. In this meeting she formally declares a breakdown in the department's financial situation. The very act of declaring such a commitment has shifted the situation from reaction to the realm of commitment and forward movement.

The fourth element involves learning the skill of distinguishing fact from interpretation. The leader of the conversation will ask questions like "What exactly has happened that is causing us to assess that now there is a problem?" or "What are the facts of the matter, as opposed to the interpretations we have?" In this process, the actual problem that needs to be resolved often changes form. What initially looked like a problem in accuracy or timeliness of reporting billing information may turn out to be more fruitfully resolved as a breakdown in the relationship between the therapists and their supervisors about treatment philosophies.

Once the facts have been established, the manager directs the inquiry with a question, such as "What are the commitments that we have made in the past, and have these particular facts occurred for us as a problem?"

This question lets the problem or "slowdown" become an opportunity to renew the commitments of the organization rather than a chance to have the individual, organization, or commitment be invalidated. Of course, there is always the possibility that upon scrutiny, we see that we are no longer actually committed to those things we once were, and the situation becomes an opportunity to design more appropriate commitments. Either way, the person, team, or group is empowered.

The fifth element is learning to use the breakdown as an opportunity for innovation and continuous quality improvement. After checking in on the commitments in the background, the manager then asks a very important question: "Given the facts and the commitments, *what is missing?*" This seemingly minor semantic shift from asking "What's wrong?" or "Who's to blame?" or "Why did this happen?" to asking "What is missing?" opens a whole new universe of thinking. "What's missing?" leads to dialog about what is possible. *The problem is now the doorway to innovation.*

For instance, we observed a treatment team beginning to implement outcome-oriented rehabilitation planning, when the weekly case conference format became confusing and unwieldy. The old goal flow sheets used to document the planning meeting process were no longer functional. As the confusion mounted, the case manager's immediate reaction was "Oh, no. This is so classic. We try something new and it never works."

The team automatically began to blame the case manager for not being "good enough" to make the meeting run smoothly. Then the case manager noticed how nonproductive this conversation was and set up a time and place to address the situation. In that meeting, the case manager declared a breakdown in documentation. As they delved into the facts, the team saw that they could be more empowered if the breakdown were declared in the area of team commitment to implementing the new planning mode. They reaffirmed their commitment to outcome-oriented planning and to effective team conferences. As the team moved through the process toward the element focusing on "what was missing," they came up with some new insights about the goal setting process.

The sixth element of the process to manage "moments of truth" is to make promises and requests that will have the team be, once again, in action toward its goals. At the conclusion of the meeting in the situation described above, two staff members volunteered to revise the goal flow sheet so that it was clearly related to outcome goals. They also identified additional actions in goal setting and display of goals in document form, which resulted in a reduction in the time the team needed to spend in conference on this issue. Finally, the team declared a breakthrough in partnership for having the new system work.

After implementing the actions, the team discovered an additional bonus. Having expedited the goal setting and tracking process, they were able to spend more time sharing clinical insights, thus building team morale.

Skills to Build

- Frame the most useful breakdown out of the multiplicity of breakdowns that could be declared, and then be able readily to reframe it, if a more empowering breakdown to declare is identified.
- Conducting successful meetings when people are upset.
- Discerning fact from interpretation.
- Being patient.

Practices

- Formally declare breakdowns.
- Record elements of the breakdown management process, such as what's missing or possible or commitments for action.
- Use a flip chart to make the process a public one.

A TRANSFORMATIONAL MANAGER'S TOOLBOX

Truly powerful organizations, individuals, or teams are those which have the ability to take an idea and make it real, quickly. The principles of transformational management described here form the core of a method to accelerate movement along the continuum from possibility to reality. We conclude this introduction to the discipline of transformational management with a description of a few of the practical tools that have been developed, to manage according to the principles of the discipline.

Purpose and Intended Results

One of the most useful tools of transformational management is to create clear statements of both purpose and intended results for meetings, projects, work processes, or even social events. This practice forces the person accountable for the action to confront why this expenditure of energy should happen and how he or she will know whether it worked or not.

By *purpose* we mean the overarching intent, the direction, the context of the matter under consideration. A purpose statement should be clear and large enough in scope to include all that the author intends to occur from the action being designed. A purpose statement answers the questions, Why are we doing this? What is the point of this? What is being served by this action/event/meeting? The purpose statement is a tool for discovering whether the conversation, project, or other is on track: that is, Are we on purpose or not?

Intended results are statements of measurable outcomes that the meeting, project, or other is designed to produce. Since it is an orientation, a purpose can go on and on. An intended result is finite; it happened or it did not. An example of a statement of purpose and intended results from a management team retreat follows:

Purpose

To empower ourselves to be effective managers, leaders, and colleagues in the midst of uncertainty and change.

Intended Results

- To have reviewed the theory and practice of dialog.
- To have clarified what is so about the organization's performance in 1994, and about the current internal and external factors in our business environment today.
- To have resolved any current breakdowns and to create alignment on the key objectives for the Q4 1994 management agenda.
- To have strengthened our relationship as a team.

The act of creating statements of purpose and intended results is a way of stating commitments clearly. It puts the person (or people) accountable for the action at risk for a specific outcome. It is a tool that highlights the future. It is an articulation of a future that *could be* if the action proceeds as intended.

When a meeting, for example, has a clear purpose and intended results, the future for which it exists is clear in advance. This will shift how the meeting occurs for the participants and allow for much more powerful and effective meetings. It gives the participants something to align on in advance (and modify, if necessary) so that all are able to "own" the meeting. It gives the group something to refer to at the meeting's conclusion, to discover whether the meeting has been effective.

Priority Documents

Another simple and effective technique for sustaining commitments over time is to create documents that state what the current priorities are for the department, team, individual, or organization. Priorities documents work best when created in partnership with those who will be accountable for the work of accomplishing them.

To call out something as a priority does not imply that it is the only thing that will be done, rather that it is an important thing to be done. When a group is clear on what its priorities are for the whole organization, subgroups and individuals can be more clear on what their priorities should be.

A priority is a chunk of work large enough to affect the outcome of the management unit materially. It will contain many tasks and actions necessary for its accomplishment. The art of creating priorities lies in part in being able to put into language the "large chunks." These documents should list a few priorities, not be a huge laundry list of everything that needs to be done in the organization.

A priority should be stated in a way that is measurable in time. There should be one person who has asked for accountability for its accomplishment, and whose accountability is public. To be accountable for the priority does not mean that individual will do all the work to achieve it.

A priorities document should be regularly referred to and updated. What was or was not accomplished is addressed and acknowledged, and new promises or key objectives take the place of the ones just completed. The actions necessary for the project's accomplishment remain in a public forum until they are completed in this manner.

For example, in Bob's rehabilitation program, the management team developed a comprehensive plan to transform the rehabilitation service into a seamless continuum of care. The purpose, intended results, quarterly objectives, and monthly and weekly priorities follow.

Rehabilitation Unit Continuum of Care Project

Purpose

To provide a seamless continuum of care for all patients requiring rehabilitation in our hospital system.

Intended Results

1. All patients admitted will receive a rehabilitation plan that crosses all levels of care required.
2. There will be no gap in continuity when the patient is transferred from inpatient to outpatient.
3. Critical pathways, treatment protocols, and documentation will be consistent throughout the service system.

Quarterly Objective

Rehabilitation plans for all patients admitted will be written from outcome targets, to include functional area goals for inpatient, outpatient, and home care as appropriate (see Exhibit 10–1).

Monthly Priorities

These tools became fully integrated into the way the department worked together. Action tracking sheets were input into the computer system, so that the management team could support one another in priority management and goal achievement. All staff were able to see the project in progress because their staff meeting, individual supervision, and task force activities were coordinated. A project progress chart was maintained on the staff office wall and a project notebook was kept at each nursing station.

Physical Space Management

Every aspect of a work environment communicates. An area often overlooked by managers is the importance of the physical environment in enhancing team spirit and performance. Transformational managers assess the work environment to see whether it is promoting the nonphysical values they are committed to keeping present. Without any expenditure on new carpets, paint, or furniture, an enormous impact can be made by simply attending to the quality of the physical environment: is it a hindrance, is it neutral, or is it a positive force for accomplishment?

When assessing the physical environment some of the following questions can be considered:

- Is this space cluttered? Are there things here that do not need to be here?
- Is this space conscious? Does it show evidence that someone has thoughtfully set it up for a purpose?
- Is this space complete? Are things put away, thrown away, or labeled in a way that indicates the next action for them?
- Is this space workable? Can we do what we need to do here? Do we have what we need to accomplish our work?
- Is this space "owned"? Are we relating to it as our space and managing it responsibly and deliberately?

A key variable in physical space management is to attend to what is being displayed there. A transformational manager asks himself or herself, "What are the signs, posters, charts, etc., that will keep us focused on the key variables that spell success?" Displays in this context might be lively signs promoting the marketing campaign, regularly updated charts that display progress toward goals and identify areas in the organization that need attention or graphs that track performance over time.

Exhibit 10–1 Continuum of Care Project Monthly Priorities

Project Priorities: March 1995

Monthly Priority: **Accountable**
1. Complete rehabilitation planning format   Mary Smith
2. Write standardized functional area goals   John Baird
   for TBI, SCI, CVA
3. Complete outpatient and home care training   Laura Williams
   in outcome-oriented rehabilitation planning
4. Design first phase of new Information System   Bruce Johnson
   software

CONCLUSION

Outcome-oriented rehabilitation is the appropriate strategy for an era of managed care and capitation. The focus on precise outcomes for a set cost is an obvious match to the economic realities dictated by the trends in health care economics. By giving staff and managers access to *being*, keeping them focused on the future, complete with the past, and in action in the present, transformational management can be a powerful tool to be used in service of meeting the twin challenges of cost reduction and quality improvement in rehabilitation medicine. When a breakthrough is needed to survive and prosper, technology for generating and sustaining breakthroughs is indicated.

In this chapter we have presented the elements of a methodology for managing to cause breakthrough outcomes. This methodology focuses on managing aspects of work that traditional management does not usually address, that is, how the design of thinking and awareness shapes action. The principles of transformational management can, when applied in the appropriate situations, give individuals, teams, and organizations access to sustained high performance.

Principles

- **Context:** To cause a breakthrough in results, shift the context for action.
- **Possibility:** The present is caused by the future.
- **Completion:** To create a new future, first release the grip of the past.
- **Listening:** The nature of the attention we give a situation, person or event, determines how it will occur for us, and how we will respond to it.
- **Speaking:** Commitments clearly expressed support sustained high performance.
- **Breakdowns**: Successful outcomes are based on well-handled breakdowns.

This chapter is an introduction to a subtle discipline. The principles are simple. Their impact can be profound. We encourage your experimentation with these principles and tools, testing them against the only true measure of the validity of an approach: the outcomes you are able to produce while using it.

The authors wish to thank Werner Erhard whose classes and seminars we have attended and whose ideas helped form many of the concepts articulated above.

REFERENCE
1. Whiteside, J. *The Phoenix Agenda: Power to Transform Your Workplace.* Essex Junction, Vt: Oliver Wight; 1994.

SUGGESTED READINGS
Goss, T, Pascale, R, and Athos, A. "The Reinvention Roller Coaster." *Harvard Business Review.* Nov/Dec; 1993.

Pascarella, P. DiBianca, V. and Gioja, L. "The Power of Responsibility." *Industry Week.* Dec; 1988.

Selman, J. and DiBianca, V. "Contextual Management: Applying the Art of Dealing Creatively with Change." *Management Review.* September; 1983.

Feinstein, D. "Breaking Out of the Box: A Crash Course in Paradigm Thinking." *Benchmark Magazine.* Fall; 1989.

Argryis, C. "Good Communication That Blocks Learning." *Harvard Business Review.* July/August; 1994.

Fittipaldi, B. "New Listening: Key to Organizational Transformation." In: *When the Canary Stops Singing: Women's Perspectives on Transforming Business,* ed. Barrentine, P. San Francisco: Berrett-Koehler; 1993.

Senge, P. *The Fifth Discipline: Mastering the Five Practices of the Learning Organization.* New York: Doubleday; 1990.

Senge, P. et al. *The Fifth Discipline Fieldbook.* New York: Doubleday; 1994.

Wheatley, M. *Leadership and the New Science.* San Francisco: Berrett-Koehler; 1992.

Chapter 11

Outcome-Based Sales and Marketing: A Partnership Approach

Paul A. Repicky, PhD, MA/LS, MAT, and Brian D. Vervynck

Objectives

- To examine how changes in health care have impacted sales and marketing in rehabilitation.
- To contrast traditional and outcome-based sales.
- To provide specific guidelines for developing strategic partnerships.
- To present methods for growing partnership relationships.

INTRODUCTION

The purpose of this chapter is to examine how the significant and ongoing changes in the U.S. health care industry have dramatically impacted the strategies and tactics required for selling and marketing products and services to that industry. We will begin by contrasting traditional sales and marketing approaches with the rationale for an outcome-based partnership strategy. This will be followed by specific guidelines for developing strategic partnerships with customers. Finally, we will present methods for maintaining and growing the partner relationship using feedback from ongoing assessment mechanisms.

CHARACTERISTICS OF THE NEW SELLING ENVIRONMENT IN THE HEALTH CARE MARKETPLACE

The Changing Health Care System

The U.S. health care industry is undergoing fundamental and significant reform driven by two primary factors. The first is the high and rising cost of health care services. The responsibility for managing these costs rests with the providers and payers. The second is that many Americans either have no health insurance or are not covered for catastrophic illness.

In response to these issues, the insurance industry/payers are promoting the concept of managed care, which bases payment for health care services on the following criteria:

- Medical need
- Medical appropriateness
- Cost-effectiveness

The providers' response is to develop organized delivery systems (ODSs) that will provide efficient, cost-effective services to contracted patient populations.

Managed Care

Managed care is the payer's response to today's high utilization and cost of health care. It represents a reorganization in the way health care services are structured, financed, and delivered. In essence, the payer has taken a supervisory role over the financing and reimbursement of health care in an attempt to manage what kind of patient care they finance/reimburse. Although managed care has been evolving over the past several years with varying degrees of success in different geographic markets, this concept is being adopted at an accelerated pace.

The impact of managed care in the marketplace varies considerably by geographic region. Regardless of the region, however, the major areas of impact will be the following:

- Financial
- Clinical
- Organizational

Since the mid-1980s, tremendous pressure has been directed to health plans to gain some control over rising health care costs. In response, health plans have developed cost containment procedures and programs. The typical model used by health plans today includes a contracted panel of physicians, hospitals, and ancillary providers. Discounted fee-for-service arrangements are negotiated from contracted providers in exchange for inclusion in the health plan's network. Utilization review is used to control inpatient hospital utilization and certain high-cost ancillary services. Case management is commonly used to help coordinate care for costly catastrophic, chronic, or high-risk conditions. Other cost containment techniques include claims review, utilization review, preadmission certification, concurrent or continued stay review, retrospective review, discharge planning, health maintenance organizations (HMOs), and preferred provider organizations (PPOs).

In an effort to contain costs, many health plans are now moving to replace their current "discounted fee-for-service model" with a prepaid or capitated system of health care financing. Under capitation, providers are at risk to control costs and utilization. They contract with a health plan to provide comprehensive service to a group of enrollees. The provider then receives a flat payment per enrollee (usually a per member per month fee). If the cost of care is more than the amount received, the provider loses money. If the cost of care is less, the provider makes money. In order to encourage physicians to control costs for specialty, hospital, and/or ancillary services, a *risk pool* is usually established. In short, capitation changes all care giving from a revenue center to a cost center.

The primary clinical impact of managed care will be a focus on outcomes through the adoption of "care paths" or protocols. In order to achieve consistent outcomes it will be necessary to follow care paths. Practice variation is a large part of outcome and cost differentiation.

The primary organizational impact of managed care is increased aggregation of providers and services into organized delivery systems (ODSs). An ODS may include physicians, payers, hospitals, home care suppliers, and ancillary providers. They need administrative services and a patient care coordination process that facilitate interaction among physicians.

The supervisory process is becoming internalized into the provider system, rather than resting with the payer, who will be very busy handling the administration. And these can continue to grow in size by successively adding components and/or merging with other ODSs.

Hospitals, physicians, insurers, and employers are rapidly developing new products and delivery systems to compete for the managed care business. The following are permutations of managed care offerings in today's marketplace: HMOs, PPOs, exclusive provider organizations (EPOs), direct purchase contracting (partnering), physician-hospital organizations (PHOs), integrated systems, and managed indemnity programs.

Providers are at varying levels in their readiness to enter the managed care environment. Practice integration models exist across a wide range. The following models range from least integrated to most integrated: solo practice, shared lease/staff, PPO, Independent Practice Association (IPA), group practice without walls, integrated medical group practice.

Impact on the Selling Environment

Health care reform impacts the sales environment dramatically. First, while the number of potential customers is decreasing, their individual size is increasing. That is, with the development of ODSs, purchasing decisions may involve representatives from several areas of the organization (e.g., clinical, financial, administrative). And each of these parties will have its own unique needs and issues on the purchase of a new product or service. Thus, the sales process will be more complex and will take longer.

> For example, a typical customer for home care services may be Beta Health Plans, a medium-sized payer that includes a PPO product and an HMO product. The key decision makers and influencers would include the medical director, the director of case management, and the director of provider relations. Each of these individuals will have different needs, concerns, and perspectives that must be addressed. These will include issues of clinical appropriateness and effectiveness, implementation, impact on various provider groups, and financial impact.

Second, any product or service sold to managed care must meet the criteria of medical appropriateness, clinical effectiveness, and cost-effectiveness. Given the intense pressure to lower the cost of health care, the latter will be of utmost importance.

Third, the ongoing changes in the players and the relationships create a dynamic environment that may breed uncertainty about the decision process and who is responsible for what.

In summary, selling in this new environment will require *more sophis-ticated, strategic, high-level sales expertise.* The environment is dynamic, with increased pressure on pricing and demonstrating outcomes. Because of the increased aggregation of providers, the "customer" is a more complex, multilayered entity.

WHAT IS OUTCOME-BASED SALES/MARKETING?

The Traditional Role of Sales and Marketing

Traditional sales approaches tend to be "transactional" in nature. The primary, overriding goal of the salesperson is to close a sale. The focus is on what the seller has to do to get the customer to agree to buy. Although many techniques are used to make it appear otherwise, ultimately sales-people focus on their own business needs.

During a sales call, this approach is characterized by a rather one-sided conversation, dominated by the salesperson. Much of the "discussion" revolves around the presentation of the features, advantages, and benefits of the product/service with the salesperson trying to make these "fit" the customer's needs. There is little attempt to enter into a true problem-solving dialog or to customize solutions for any given customer. At some point, the salesperson tries to "close" the sale by asking for a commitment to buy. This attempt is usually met with outright objections or unexplained noncommitment. In response to objections, the general tactic is to try to convince the customers to change their mind by telling them why their perception is incorrect, why they really need the product/service, that they don't really understand how it can help them, or something similar. The more skilled salesperson attempts to identify customer needs that their product/service can meet and explore these needs in some depth to strengthen their case further.

As an example of this type of sales behavior, consider the following dialog between a real estate agent and a couple interested in buying a home.

AGENT: Good afternoon. How can I help you?

BUYERS: Hello, my wife and I are looking for a home.

AGENT: Wonderful! What is your price range?

BUYERS: $225,000 to $250,000.

AGENT: Well, let me show you some houses you might like. Here's the first one, and although it's $300,000, I'm sure a couple of your stature will find it appealing.

BUYERS: Well, it looks nice from the outside, but it is beyond our budget.

AGENT: I understand but, since we're here, let's take a look anyway. I'm sure you'll really love this house; it's my favorite! Just look at all the room you have here, including 4 bedrooms, enough for several children.

BUYERS: Oh, we don't have any children.

AGENT: That's OK, you're still young and it never hurts to plan ahead, right? Let me show you the gourmet kitchen. It has all the latest features to enable you to create some outstanding home-cooked meals that everyone loves.

BUYERS: Well, we both have busy careers and eat almost all our meals out.

AGENT: Then let me show you the lap pool; it's fabulous. It's fully heated with solar panels and provides a convenient workout facility.

BUYERS: Although we both keep in good physical shape, I prefer to run and my husband lifts weights. Neither of us swims.

Clearly, from this brief dialog some basic sales patterns are emerging. The agent is doing most of the talking and is trying to sell something he *thinks* the buyers want. The agent isn't asking what the buyers really want in a home; he's more preoccupied with what he has to sell them. Initial questions the agent might have asked include "Do you have any children?" "What, to you, are the most important features of a home?" "What type of neighborhood would you like to live in?" "How long do you intend to live in the home?" "Do you have any hobbies, such as woodworking, gardening, or music?" All of these would help the agent identify specific homes that meet the buyers' criteria and allow the agent to emphasize the appropriate features of each home they see.

Equally important to the actual content of the sales call conversation is how the customer *feels*. In fact, the basis of any buying decision is a feeling, an emotion. Unfortunately, the general perception of salespeople and the sales profession is not positive. Although salespeople may be seen as friendly, outgoing, quick-witted individuals, customers often sense some superficiality in the relationship. This feeling is expressed in the notion "They are just trying to sell me something." In general, salespeople approach selling as an adversarial relationship. In their minds they "win" if they get the order and the way the customer feels really doesn't matter very much. While customers may feel that the salesperson is interested in them and their needs, they know this will last only so long as there is a sale to be made. After that, any sense of relationship or caring dissipates rapidly. Interestingly, people generally do not like to be sold something; however, they do like to buy. That's the paradox within the traditional sales environment.

Partnerships: A New Relationship between Buyer and Seller

In contrast to these traditional sales approaches, the primary goal of partnership strategies is to develop a trusting and enduring relationship with the customer. Through the relationship, the partners truly work together to solve problems, meet needs, and work to achieve mutually agreeable outcomes. Partnership development specialists do not have preconceived notions that they "know best." Proper solutions are only arrived at after a thorough understanding of *each other's* businesses and how they can *jointly* develop alternatives. The partners use all their available resources, as required, to meet the needs of the partnership. In essence, the parties function as if they are partners in the same business. Clearly, this collegial attitude represents a fundamental shift. The partners have the sense that "we" are working together to solve problems and enhance each other's business rather than feeling that one partner is trying to get the other to buy something. With this nonadversarial approach, all the partners are winners.

In this context, a partnership is defined as a mutually beneficial and enduring relationship founded on trust, honesty, and commonality of goals. The partnership relationship is characterized by longevity, change, and growth. Trust is the fundamental underpinning of the relationship; without it a partnership cannot be developed. In a more traditional approach trust is gained on the golf course, at dinners, and so forth. In developing a partnership, trust is gained by demonstration of business knowledge and the ability to provide consistent and reliable service.

Creation of a partnership requires that each party develop a broad and deep knowledge and understanding of the other's business. With this understanding the partners can creatively examine new ways to expand the relationship. Expanding the relationship requires flexibility of both partners, who must be willing to examine the way they do business and, at times, modify their methods to enhance the effectiveness and success of the partnership. Both partners must be constantly alert to opportunities to grow the partnership.

A summary of our experience in developing a partnership with Company X will illustrate specific applications of this concept. In our initial discussions with Company X we made it clear that we were looking for a long-term relationship/partnership and gained their agreement that this goal was in concert with their plans. The scope of our initial contract was to assess their existing sales organization. Although we agreed on a fixed-term, consulting contract, both parties clearly understood that, depending on our performance, the relationship could be extended for a much longer period.

In performing this assessment, we conducted extensive interviews of all the key personnel and collected information from a variety of sources. This process served three purposes: Our analysis and recommendations confirmed their suspicions regarding the quality of their sales organization; we gained, in a short period, a working knowledge of their business and the personalities of the key personnel in the organization; and, through our analysis, we demonstrated a portion of our capabilities. We had succeeded in developing strong credibility and trust.

Consequently, we were asked to expand our commitment to developing their sales organization; that would necessitate full-time involvement of one of our senior executives, and we agreed. It is noteworthy that from that point on our relationship has been based on a handshake; there is no written contract between us and Company X. While this arrangement may not be the most prudent from a legal perspective, it clearly demonstrates the strength of the partnership and the high level of trust of both partners.

As we became more involved in our partner's business we identified needs of Company X in the areas of training development and delivery, conceptualization of new business strategies, and facilitation of strategic planning meetings. We have provided considerable services in these areas. All of these are value-added: that is, they were provided as part of the partnership arrangement, at no extra charge. These efforts have enabled us to expand our value to Company X and further enhance our partnership. Our challenge was to strive constantly to bring value to the partnership. Clearly, our focus was not on closing new business/making immediate sales but, rather, in building the relationship. As a consequence, Company X has recommended our services to other companies, actively supports our sales to those companies, and is positioning us with them as they expand the scope of their business activity.

The development of a partnership requires specific, high-level sales skills. In fact, the difference is so significant that we can replace the term *salesperson* with *partnership development specialist* and the term *customer* with *partner*. This process requires a significant shift in focus from the interests of the partnership development specialist to those of the partner. When this shift is effectively accomplished, partners feel, not that they have "been sold" something, but that they are participating in a process with a genuinely interested, trusted organization that will enhance their respective businesses.

This principle is illustrated through another example. We were contracted by Company Y to develop strategic partnerships with large organizations who would use their service. Upon initiation of one such partnership it became clear that successful implementation of Company Y's services would require a significant administrative effort and ongoing sales/service activities within the corporate office of the new partner. To assure a smooth transition and to facilitate communication and continuing support within that large organization, we elected to place one of Company Y's field service representatives on-site at the partner's corporate offices, on a regular, part-time basis. This move was perceived as a value-added service, with no additional cost to the partner organization and has been an effective strategy for development of the partnership.

Shift to a Behavioral Outcome Approach

At the heart of the partnership development process is a focus on outcomes. Outcomes are defined in terms of observable, measurable behaviors of the partner that ultimately satisfy the needs of all parties. This level of focus on outcomes represents a fundamental conceptual shift in the psychological basis of sales. Whereas salespeople have generally been more concerned with how they would make their presentation, what issues they would and would not like to discuss, and what they would say in response to certain objections, the partnership development specialist focuses more on what the potential partner is doing, that is, his behavior. In fact, the most important element is not what the partnership development specialist does; it's what the potential partner does.

The following are sample sales objectives that specify the customer's behavior. The customer will

- agree to a follow-up appointment to explore in greater detail the product/service being offered,
- assist you in setting up an inservice for the clinical staff,
- introduce you to a key decision maker in the organization,
- agree to implement a 30-day evaluation of the product/service,
- request a proposal for our services,
- commit to support, at the next board meeting, the purchase of the product/service,
- arrange for a technical review of the product by their engineers.

Certainly this emphasis on objectives does not imply that what the partnership development specialist (PDS) does is not important; it is just secondary. The behavior of the PDS is critical because it influences the behavior of the partner. No matter how eloquent the presentation or how logical the argument, however, it is of little use if the partner does not respond positively, as intended by the PDS.

Thus, outcome-based selling means a focus on results. These behavioral outcomes are the basis for sales call planning and evaluation of progress. They can also be used as a basis for compensation.

STRATEGIES AND TACTICS FOR DEVELOPING PARTNERSHIPS

Targeting

Targeting is the process of identifying and then ranking potential partners for a business. Effective targeting is critical because it maximizes the utilization of partnership development resources. Through a concentration of efforts the partnership development process can be accelerated.

The criteria for identifying potential partners may include any number of factors including appropriate fit for products/services offered, potential value of the relationship to both parties, and geographic location. Once potential partners have been identified, specific criteria should be applied to help prioritize them. A most important criterion is a determination of the current level of your partnership relationship. The Partnership Assessment Scale (PAS) (Exhibit 11–1) defines four levels of a partnership relationship. Once the level of the current relationship has been determined, it forms the basis for developing a strategic plan for growing the partnership, for sequencing partnership development objectives, and for evaluating success. Additional criteria for prioritizing potential partners may include their belief in the value of products/services of the type provided, their current utilization of competitive products/services, their existing relationships with decision makers or influencers, and their relationship with other potential/current partners.

For example, if you were selling computer software that enabled physicians to create a totally paperless office environment and to connect with various ancillary services such as laboratories, pharmacies, and home health care agencies, you might proceed as follows:

Exhibit 11–1 Partnership Assessment Scale (PAS)

LEVEL I
> The potential partner has no, or limited, knowledge of your products/services and no understanding of how they might meet their needs

LEVEL II
> The potential partner has limited-to-extensive knowledge/understanding of your products/services and may use some of them, occasionally

LEVEL III
> The potential partner regularly uses some/most of the appropriate products/services you offer and clearly understands their application to their business

LEVEL IV
> The partner is actively involved in analyzing your product/service offerings and working with you to improve them and strengthen the relationship

---

- Identify the types of organizations that might have a need for this product (e.g., managed care organizations).
- Identify specific target locations based on population size, concentration of managed care organizations, and proximity to your distribution/service centers.
- Select specific organizations within those target locations on the basis of criteria such as willingness to adopt new technologies, leadership stature in the medical community, strong clinical reputation, a well-managed organization, and one that aggressively seeks ways to be more effective in health care delivery.

Collecting Background Information

Accurate, comprehensive background information on your potential partners is absolutely critical to your success in developing a partnership relationship. The more information you have and the better you understand your partner, the better your chances of creating an effective partnership development strategy. By doing this research you help to prevent the common objection "You don't really understand my situation." It also allows you to anticipate potential areas of concern for your partner and to develop solutions in advance.

Specifically, you need to determine everything you can about the organization, such as the products/services they offer; their market, their current customers; their business volume; the advantages and disadvantages of their products/services; the advantages and disadvantages of their competitors' products/services; the needs/problems of the organization; the organization's culture/personality; their financial position; their existing relationships or partnerships with other organizations; how/whether they currently fulfill their need for the types of products/services you offer; and the advantages and disadvantages of their current solutions to the needs addressed by your products/services.

It is also important to identify the key decision makers and those who influence them. You'll need to know their position in the organization, their span of control, their relationship to other decision makers and influencers, their specific needs/problems, and their personalities and how they prefer to be treated by potential partners.

A variety of techniques can be used to obtain this information. As a general principle, you should try to gather as much of this information as possible when you are *not* in direct contact with the key decision makers.

You should reserve that time for moving the relationship forward while demonstrating your in-depth knowledge of their business. One source of information is documentation such as quarterly and annual reports, organization newsletters, advertising, and marketing literature. Another source is individuals in the organization who are not decision makers, but are in midlevel management positions.

Strategic Partnership Development Planning

The complexity of the new selling environment requires a strategic approach to partnership development. Simply put, employing a strategic approach means analyzing the background information to target the most appropriate potential partners, determining overall development goals and time lines for each potential partner, developing a set of specific objectives that will lead to accomplishment of each goal, and designing specific strategies and tactics to accomplish those objectives.

The ongoing record of this activity is documented in the Strategic Partner Development Plan (Exhibit 11–2), which summarizes the key information and progress toward partnership development. While this document provides a critical, overall picture, it does not include specific strategies and tactics for partner development. This information is recorded in the Annual and Quarterly Partnership Development Plans (Exhibits 11–3 and 11–4). In addition, specific planning information and results are documented in the Partnership Call Report (Exhibit 11–5).

These planning documents are designed to reflect the concepts of outcome-based strategic partnership development. It is essential that these concepts be constantly reinforced in every step of the process because, more than a set of techniques, they are a way of thinking.

Each of these documents includes objectives. These objectives are absolutely critical. Each is a statement of a specific, measurable partner behavior: that is, what the partner will do as a result of the event. They serve as an objective, demonstrable basis for evaluating your progress with each partner.

Direct Sales Skills

First and foremost, the ability to build relationships and a sense of trust is absolutely critical to partnership development. Trust is necessary

Exhibit 11–2 Strategic Partnership Development Plan

1. Background Information

    Partner: _____

    Address: _____

    Phone: (   )_____ FAX: (   )_____

    Description:

    _____
    _____
    _____

    Decision Makers/Titles (background, personality type, needs/concerns, reports to):

    _____
    _____
    _____

    Decision Influencers/Titles:

    _____
    _____
    _____

    Scope/Capabilities (history, market, capabilities, etc.)

    _____
    _____
    _____

PAS Rating: I II III IV

Rationale for PAS Rating:

_____
_____
_____

2. Problems/Needs

_____
_____
_____

3. Implications of Needs

_____
_____
_____

continues

Exhibit 11–2 continued

4. Specific Solutions to Needs

_____

_____

_____

5. Objections

_____

_____

_____

6. Objectives Achieved to Date

_____

_____

_____

7. Future Objectives

_____

_____

_____

8. Call History

   a. Date

      (1) Location

      (2) Attendees

      (3) Follow-up Actions (who/what/when)

   b. Date

      (1) Location

      (2) Attendees

      (3) Follow-up Actions (who/what/when)

Exhibit 11–3 Annual Partnership Development Plan

Year:_____   Partner: _____

Objectives Achieved in Previous Year:
_____
_____
_____

Objectives for This Year:
_____
_____
_____

Strategy:
_____
_____
_____

Current PAS Rating: I   II   III   IV

Projected PAS Rating for Next Year: I   II   III   IV

Projected Monthly Milestones for Achieving New PAS Rating:
Month 1 _____
Month 2 _____
Month 3 _____
Month 4 _____
Month 5 _____
Month 6 _____
Month 7 _____
Month 8 _____
Month 9 _____
Month 10 _____
Month 11 _____
Month 12 _____

Comments/Notes of Special Interest:
_____

Exhibit 11–4 Quarterly Partnership Development Plan

Quarter:_____   Partner: _____

Objectives Achieved in Previous Quarter:

_____
_____
_____

Objectives for This Quarter:

_____
_____
_____

Strategy:

_____
_____
_____

Current PAS Rating: I   II   III   IV

Projected PAS Rating for Next Quarter: I   II   III   IV

Projected Weekly Milestones for Achieving New PAS Rating:

Week 1 _____
Week 2 _____
Week 3 _____
Week 4 _____
Week 5 _____
Week 6 _____
Week 7 _____
Week 8 _____
Week 9 _____
Week 10 _____
Week 11 _____
Week 12 _____

Comments/Notes of Special Interest:

_____

Exhibit 11–5 Partnership Call Report

Date:_____   Partner: _____

Appointment Time:_____   Actual Meeting Time:_____

Location: _____

Contact (Partner Representatives): _____

Partnership Development Representatives:_____

Purposes:

    1. _____

    2. _____

Objectives (behavioral statements):

    1. _____

    2. _____

    3. _____

    4. _____

    5. _____

Tactics (Presentation, questioning, discussion, sales/marketing aids):

    1. _____

    2. _____

    3. _____

    4. _____

    5. _____

continues

Exhibit 11–5 continued

Post-Call Summary

Results:

Objective #1: _____

Objective #2: _____

Objective #3: _____

Objective #4: _____

Objective #5: _____

PAS Rating: I   II   II   IV

Notes:

1. _____

2. _____

3. _____

Next Actions:

Item	Resources	Date Completed
1.		
2.		
3.		
4.		

because a partnership relationship requires that the partners reveal significant information about their business strategies and tactics, their products/services, and their personnel. To develop, maintain, and enhance such a relationship require skills in communication, listening skills, behavioral flexibility, and influence.

While building a relationship, it is also necessary to uncover, clarify, and expand issues and to influence your partner's behavior. Telling or coercing people in what they should do is not an effective way to create partnerships and does not work long-term. The most powerful verbal tool for accomplishing both these objectives is questions. Through the skillful use of questions you can get potential partners to provide information, consider alternative perspectives on an issue, and recommend solutions without creating a feeling of "being sold" in your partner. They make the decisions, but through your efforts at building a relationship you have earned the right to influence those decisions. For this reason, questioning skills are undoubtedly the most important sales skill area in the current environment.

The third major skill area is in developing and presenting solutions that will meet your partner's needs. Effective implementation of such solutions may require great flexibility. You may have to consider ways that you can reconfigure your product/service to meet their needs. Also, as solutions are presented, it is common for objections to be raised. There is a finite number of issues, questions, concerns that partners will have, however, about any product/service, and these can be addressed effectively by using any of several techniques.

First, as you begin to understand the concerns your partners may have about your product/service, you can alleviate many of them by establishing up-front specific expectations of performance and explaining the rationale behind them. Through this process it is even possible to turn potential objections into perceived benefits.

Second, you should validate their objections rather than argue about them. Everyone has a unique perspective on any given issue, and in terms of that perspective, the person is right! When an objection arises you should

- ask questions to clarify the person's perspective/reasoning,
- ask questions that will allow him or her to look at the issue from a different perspective,
- never contradict the person's perspective; people do not like to be told they are wrong.

Third, when an objection is raised, you can redirect attention toward a solution. For example, you might ask, "I appreciate your concern about this issue and I was just wondering what would happen if we could alleviate it completely in a very short time?" If this statement is made with sincerity and honesty, you should be able to redirect attention from complaining to focusing on development of a solution.

Fourth, in response to an objection you might try to change the meaning or context of the objectionable event. To accomplish this change, you should ask yourself the following questions:

- "What else could this event mean that would have a positive value?"
- "In what context would this event have positive value?"

This technique will only be successful to the extent that it helps the person feel better emotionally.

Fifth, you can attempt to make any objection the final objection. To accomplish this, simply ask, "Is X the only thing holding you back? If we could handle X, would you agree to proceed to the next step?" This approach will serve two objectives. It should get all concerns out on the table so you can deal with them more efficiently. Also, it implies a subtle commitment that if you handle these concerns, the person will have some obligation to move forward with you.

Sixth, you should be able to alleviate "buyer's remorse," which is an objection that occurs after the person commits to move forward. After you have achieved agreement, ask your partner to step into the future and describe all the ways that he or she will use the service/product for the next several months/year. Get the person to feel good about the decision in advance. Having this feeling will reaffirm in the buyer's mind that the decision is the right decision and cause the buyer to expect positive results.

Seventh, you will become much more effective in handling objections if you learn to eliminate feelings of rejection and failure. The key to this process is to recognize that these feelings are based on decisions we make. We all have our own rules for making these decisions, and one way to overcome these feelings is to change the rules. For example, if you define failure as, "not getting precisely the outcome you expect, when you expect it," then you are likely to experience feelings of failure quite often. If you define success, however, as "learning something useful from any outcome you achieve," then you are likely to experience more feelings of success.

Finally, using visualization techniques you can prepare yourself to respond to objections before they ever occur. People will respond more to your nonverbal cues and your voice qualities than to what you say. Through visualization practice you can become extremely effective in *how* to respond as well as *what* to say.

Partnership Agreements

Partnership agreements that describe the objectives of the partnership and the respective responsibilities of the parties, once created, serve as the basis for clarity in the partnership relationship.

These can be oral or written agreements that describe the objectives of the partnership and the respective responsibilities of the partners. In developing this understanding it is essential to assess each partner on a scale and present the appropriate mix of standardized services, in a customized package/presentation. These agreements clarify the partnership relationship.

The Strategic Partnership Plan

The heart of a partnership relationship is embodied in the strategic partnership plan. This document contains all the key elements that define and operationalize the partnership. It may include any or all of the following:

- Partnership goals—a statement of the intended global outcomes
- Organizational charts—identifying the key individuals and basic reporting relationships within the partnership, characteristics, needs, and so on
- Annual and quarterly objectives—specific objectives of the partnership, each defined by behavioral anchors, as appropriate; includes objectives now achieved to illustrate past accomplishments as well as future direction
- Obstacles to success—a listing of existing or potential roadblocks to achieving the partnership objectives
- Action plan—guided by quarterly objectives; includes strategies, tactics, action items, responsible individuals, resources required, completion dates, and description of current status for specific periods

The strategic partnership plan serves many functions. First, it formalizes or solidifies the relationship. While this type of planning and documentation activity is customary within an organization, it is even more essential in a strategic partnership because the relationship is less formal and more dynamic. Second, it is a tool that facilitates communication between the partner organizations. Third, it provides an instant status update/overview regarding the progress of the partnership. The objectives and behavioral anchors provide a checklist for assessing progress. Fourth, it serves as a guide for development of action plans because it documents effective and ineffective strategies and tactics.

NURTURING AND GROWING THE PARTNERSHIP

Defining the Partnership and Identifying Common Goals

A strategic partnership is a new and unique entity. Although it is different from a legal partnership agreement, the spirit of cooperation, mutual benefit, and working together to move toward common goals is identical in both arrangements. For purposes of this discussion we are using the term *partnership* in the nonlegal sense.

To clarify further, let's examine the defining characteristics of a strategic partnership. First, the relationship is based on mutual respect and trust. This element is absolutely essential and directly related to the success of the partnership. Certainly the development of respect and trust requires effort and skill of all partners. And, it is an ongoing, and perhaps endless process.

Second, a strategic partnership is a mutually beneficial business relationship between two or more parties (partners). The partners must determine early in the relationship that there is a commonality of interest and that they each can offer products/services that will assist their partner in their business. The products/services must meet existing needs. As an example, consider the relationships being crafted between the large indemnity payers and the various emerging companies developing health care delivery and management systems designed to "carve out" a specific, high-risk patient population and go at risk for providing care at a fixed or predetermined cost structure. The payers benefit from the relationship by off-loading their risk to an organization that specializes in providing care to those patients. In turn, the provider group enjoys a stream of patients that they can treat profitably because of their highly specialized care capabilities.

Third, generally this relationship is long-term. It takes time and effort to develop deep levels of trust and respect, to explore the many potential facets of the relationship, and to develop new or redesign existing products/services that evolve as a result of the synergy between the partner organizations.

Fourth, the parties engage in a strategic planning process in which they define common goals. This activity requires the partners to reveal their corporate philosophies, strategies, and tactics. It may also involve discussion of plans to enter new markets and the future directions of the organizations. All of this can be very sensitive and confidential information. Before discussions can take place at this level the relationship must be extremely well developed and the partners must be ready to look openly at new ideas. This process requires great flexibility of all sides. The ability to have these discussions is the ultimate test of a partnering relationship, however, and clearly has the greatest potential for positive impact on each of the partners.

Development of Internal Management Systems

The definition of roles and functions within the partnership is essential to the creation of an effective, productive relationship. This process often involves development of new relationships and implementation of new strategies and procedures.

Considerable flexibility is required to create new solutions that optimize the talents and resources of the partners. The existing infrastructure may need to be modified to accommodate the new relationship. As new roles are created, individuals may assume significant responsibilities and titles within their partner's organization. From the perspective of the customers of this partnership, these relationships may be clearly delineated or they may remain transparent. For example, it may be necessary to form a strategic partnership development team with representation from each partner organization. The team's charge would be to assess the outcomes of the current relationship and to create new directions for both organizations that have become possible because of the partnership's existence.

Information systems are the key to communication and efficiency within and between the organizations comprising the partnership. Since each organization is likely to have existing systems, the challenge will be to adopt mechanisms that can be readily implemented by all partners. In addition to the systems, for each partner the individuals and their responsibilities must be clear to their partner organization.

Finally, regular reporting mechanisms must be implemented to enhance communication and monitor progress. Reports should include, as a minimum, monthly updates indicating specific accomplishments that are keyed to quarterly and annual goals.

ASSESSMENT/EVALUATION OF PARTNER BEHAVIOR

Evaluation of Partnership Status

The status of a partnership can be assessed at any time by determining which objectives have already been achieved and which have not. These are the same objectives identified on the strategic partnership development plan. They represent the outcomes of the process. The effectiveness of the strategies and tactics relates directly to their success in producing targeted behaviors. Thus, the need for directly observable, measurable behaviors is fundamental.

It is essential to conduct periodic reviews of the partnership's progress with your partners. These reviews should include an assessment of the partnership status, goal setting, analysis of obstacles, and development of strategies and tactics for moving to the next level. The stronger the relationship, the more effective these reviews will be in enhancing the success of the partnership.

Definition of Objectives and Behavioral Anchors

The basis for assessing the development and progress of a partnership lies in the identification of specific objectives that describe the desired results. And it is particularly important that these objectives be clearly defined by "behavioral anchors" that can be observed and measured.

For example, suppose that one desired outcome was to have Department "A" within one organization "work more closely with" the partner organization. Without further refinement, it is likely that varied interpretations of "work more closely with" will exist among the individuals involved. However, answering the question "What specifically will the members of this department have to do in order for all involved to agree that they are working more closely with the partner organization?" will allow the development of specific behavioral anchors that define this outcome. The following are possible types of responses:

- John Smith will begin having weekly meetings with the partner organization for the purpose of developing and implementing joint strategies to assist John's department in creating the new service.
- Bill Jones of the partner organization will interview key potential customers and produce an analysis of the primary needs that should be met by the new service.
- The partner organization will send a representative to all service design meetings.

This list of behaviors serves to "anchor" the meaning of the term "work more closely with." As a result of this process, representatives from both organizations should be able to assess whether or not these behaviors occur.

The objectives and their respective behavioral anchors should be determined jointly by representatives from the partner organizations. This joint effort will accomplish several objectives. First, it will facilitate communication between the partners as well as a better understanding of their cultures, philosophies, and flexibility. Second, it will provide great clarity about the objectives that can be used as the basis for ongoing assessment and review by the partners. Third, it will provide the basis for development of specific action plans for both partners. The plan is developed through the assignment of responsibility for objectives and prioritization. Fourth, it assists in determining the allocation of the partnership's resources.

Joint Planning and Problem Solving

The development of common goals, objectives, and specific behaviors that define those objectives establishes the direction of the partnership. In order to achieve efficient, effective progress toward partnership goals, it is essential that the partners engage in a regular process of joint planning and problem solving. In many aspects this process is not different from traditional business planning: goals are established; milestones, strategies, and tactics are designed; and progress is monitored via regular reporting mechanisms and reviews.

The differences in a partnership involve the unique challenges and opportunities that derive from the relationship. For example, there may be a natural reluctance for partners to reveal to each other their internal weaknesses or deficiencies. Regular information flow on changes in a dynamic business environment may be difficult to achieve with a partner who does not have an on-site representative. Partners may, at least initially, be reluctant to critique their partner's performance or to offer suggestions for improvement.

On the other hand, the combined resources of the partners should facilitate problem identification and resolution, creation of new ideas and directions for the partnership, sales and marketing efforts, expansion of market share through sharing of customers, and entry into new markets as new product/service offerings are created.

For example, consider this scenario. Mr. Wilson invented a computer peripheral product designed to alleviate, and perhaps eliminate, the problem of carpal tunnel syndrome as well as associated neck and shoulder problems resulting from extensive keyboard use. Concurrently, and independently, Dr. James created a seating device designed to alleviate low back pain and improve circulation in the legs for individuals who must sit for extended periods. Both individuals wished to take their products to the marketplace but lacked the skills and capital to do so effectively. Coincidentally, a company known as "Strategic Partners, Inc." was introduced to these two individuals and their products. Taking advantage of the natural synergies between these two products, the company created a new entity, "Ergonomic Products, Inc.," and obtained the rights to market the two products. As anticipated, natural synergies emerged: Many of the customer audiences for the two products were identical: that is, office workers who sit at keyboards for extended periods. Great efficiencies were achieved in advertising, sales, and distribution of the products. Often, customers attracted by one product became customers for both. Ultimately, both products achieved enhanced market success that would have been difficult to achieve independently. And the two original inventors became close colleagues and went on to codevelop a series of successful ergonomic products for office workers.

Chapter 12

Knowledge-Based Systems in Rehabilitation: The Foundation for Outcome Achievement

Alvin McLean, Jr., PhD, Michael D. Peters, PhD, and Ann Bodin

---

Objectives

- To glimpse how outcome-based rehabilitation is done in the year 2000.
- To distinguish between data, information, and knowledge.
- To understand the different aspects of data selection, collection, and display through both theory and example.
- To present the salient steps in creating an automated data and information system.
- To present how information systems can be designed to create knowledge and to identify the six characteristics of a knowledge-based business.

REHAB 2000

James Jones is a 24-year-old male who sustained a moderately severe brain injury in a motor vehicle accident. He had a Glasgow Coma Scale score of 9 in the emergency room, a right frontoparietal contusion, a comminuted fibula-tibia fracture of the left leg, and a subcapsular hemorrhage of the liver and spleen. Mr. Jones services cellular telephones and equipment and was driving between work appointments at the time of his injury. He is single and lives with his mother, a divorced school-teacher. He has no siblings. Both his mother and employer have been supportive since his injury. He was admitted to the step-down unit of the neurosurgery department and a rehabilitation team consultation was requested. Physiatry; neuropsychology; rehabilitation nursing; occupational; physical and speech therapies; and internal case management completed *coordinated evaluations* that totaled 3 hours for all the disciplines. Each team member's evaluation focused on that person's area of expertise, and the comprehensive evaluation allowed for minimal overlap in the type of data collected by each discipline. The data are collected such that the evaluation can either be completed on a laptop computer or inputted into a personal computer (PC) from a paper-and-pencil form. Data entry takes approximately 20 minutes. These data go into *RehaSys*, an expert database system for rehabilitation service delivery. On the basis of data collected, the internal case manager is able to run a program that determines the patient's *complexity* and specifies with .90 probability how long it will take this patient to achieve an *overall outcome level I* (physiologic stability), with .85 probability how long it will take to achieve an *overall outcome level II* (physiologic maintenance), and with .80 probability how long it will take to achieve an *overall outcome level III* (home integration).

Given the data available, it is not possible to determine community integration and vocational reentry outcomes at the time of the coordinated evaluations. The standard operating procedure that this team has set forth is that any predictions below a .80 probability are too variable and should not be considered in treatment planning activities until more data are available. In addition to these overall outcome levels, the internal case manager's system also delineates the specific *target outcomes* that are required by each discipline in order for the patient to achieve the overall outcome levels I, II, and III. For example, there is a required orthopedic management outcome for physiatry that specifies how the fibula-tibia fracture must be managed. For nursing, there is a required bowel and bladder outcome, and for physical therapy, required ambulation outcomes, and for the entire team required safety management outcomes, and so forth.

Associated with each outcome is a *treatment protocol* that delineates the specific objectives of each target outcome, the procedures that should be employed to achieve each objective, how the objectives will be measured, and the criteria that will be used to determine whether the objective has been met. Prior to use, each protocol was cross-validated between clinicians for efficacy as well as resources expended to achieve criteria. The result of following this type of protocol development strategy was that each individual protocol reflected the best demonstrated practice as well as supplying standards to measure patient progress toward outcome achievement.

Finally, the system determines *length of treatment* required to accomplish the targeted outcomes and the overall outcomes. This is done by comparing the evaluation findings for Mr. Jones with those of patients with the same diagnosis and similar complexity levels who have achieved the same outcome levels and similar targeted outcomes as well as aggregating projected resource consumption from treatment protocols targeted for implementation. The administrator of the rehabilitation department can now take the data on length of stay and number of treatment sessions required by each clinician to achieve the target outcomes, factor in error variance, and determine the *case rate price* for Mr. Jones to achieve outcome levels I, II, and eventually III .

This price can then be compared to the average case rate price for all rehabilitation patients, to brain injury versus spinal cord injury, to similar brain injury patients for the prior fiscal year, to similar brain injury patient case rates for local competitor hospitals, to similar brain injury patient case rates for competitor hospitals in different regions of the country, or to similar brain injury patients within the national database. This same process will be replicated when Mr. Jones has achieved level III and is ready for community reintegration and return to his previous employer in a modified job. This is the essence of a knowledge-based rehabilitation management system that facilitates the achievement of durable clinical outcomes reliably, cost-effectively, and efficiently.

The scenario described here delineates how rehabilitation will be done in this country in the year 2000. We can vividly describe it today because a number of components of this system are already in place and their efficacy is being measured and tested currently. Chapters 3 to 6 of this book describe some of those systems. Davis and Botkin in a recent article in the *Harvard Business Review* describe the process that many businesses have gone through over the past 20 years in the movement from data to information to knowledge. Rehabilitation is going through a similar maturation at this time. The distinctions between these three processes can be illustrated in the examples that follow. Data are the basic building blocks of the "information economy" and of a "knowledge-based business." For example, the facts that Mr. Jones is 24 years of age and sustained a brain injury with a Glasgow Coma Scale score of 9, was employed as a service person, and lives with his mother are data. Information, on the other other hand, is data organized into meaningful patterns. The points regarding Mr. Jones's age, brain injury severity, and psychosocial status can be organized in a manner to calculate his overall complexity score, which is information. The conversion of this information into knowledge depends to some extent on the user. Knowledge is the application and productive use of information. For example, the rehabilitation team is able to take the data on the patient Mr. Jones, organize the data into information, and then apply this information to produce a result: outcome achievement. An even more intriguing example of knowledge is the ability to take the information regarding complexity and the information regarding the outcome level that Mr. Jones is capable of achieving and then predict the cost in dollars and resource utilization to facilitate the patient's achievement of his outcome level.

This chapter is divided into three sections: Data, Information, and Knowledge. The first section focuses on data collection: What to collect, how to measure it, and how to present it graphically to create usable information. The second section focuses on information and systems for storing and converting data into information. In the final section, the six principles of a knowledge-based business are discussed, emphasizing how these principles can be utilized in the achievement of clinical outcomes.

DATA: SELECTION, COLLECTION, AND DISPLAY

One of the purposes of the current chapter is to provide a basic introduction to data selection, collection, and display. For the purposes of this chapter, *basic* should not be taken as pejorative; as in all applied environments, there are multiple challenges to reliability of data collected. Our experience is that basic data well collected are significantly more useful than complex data collected poorly or not at all.

It should be quite evident that excluding the more standard diagnostic tests, data collection in rehabilitation has historically been open to criticism of subjectivity. Reliability and accuracy of data collection across observers have been lacking, causing problems both at the level of the patient and at the level of aggregates of patients. Lack of standard measures and reporting technologies leads to challenges of the individual clinician as well as the field as a whole. And yet, there continues, on all levels, to the adoption of more rigorous and objective measures of patient status before, during, and after clinical interventions. Opponents of objective rigor in the form of hard data collection and display often take refuge in the long enduring notion that rehabilitation is an "art" rather than a "science." It is our contention that acceptance of rehabilitation as an "art" has been due to the complexity of the task at hand where typically multiple systems are impacted by the injury and the fact that collection of data on aggregates of patients has been rare within rehabilitation. Therefore, patients are seen as heterogeneous and treatment is thus individualized.

Yet, there is clear and consistent evidence that the culture in the form of the payer, patient, and clinical research communities are increasingly unwilling to accept subjective or idiosyncratic measures of patient progress. Recognition of this is resulting in a trend away from an "art" to a "science" of rehabilitation, meaning that there have been increasing demands for data that is objective and reliable and that takes a standard and consistent format. It is interesting to note that within neurologic rehabilitation, the specialty area of neurobehavioral remediation has long relied on a scientific methodology for development and application of its interventions. An example of application of a scientific methodology is seen in Peters, Gluck, and McCormick[1] with a more broad treatment found in Pace and Nau.[2] Extension of a scientific methodology to rehabilitation at large will be of benefit to patient, provider, and payer. There are a number of clinically superb programs that have historically collected and utilized data in clinical decision making. Some of these are described in Chapters 4 through 6 in this book. The emphasis of this data collection has primarily been on functional outcome levels such as self-care, ambulation, community mobility, and medication management.

The data collection we are proposing takes the construct one step deeper to examine not just the result (independence in self-care) but how the result is achieved. Measuring the process as well as the result allows one to examine more carefully how things can be done more effectively and efficiently. It also provides a road map such that the steps can be retraced and a new route charted if the current route does not produce the intended result. For example, in the self-training protocol that we are discussing the data collected would include the criteria used to measure whether the outcome has been achieved, the detailed procedure for achieving the outcome, and the amount of resources utilized to accomplish this outcome. Setting up a system to collect these type of data allows you to have a structure for answering questions such as "Can I achieve this same result more efficiently?" "Can this result be replicated in hospital X, Y, or Z?" "If the outcome was not achieved, where in the process did the difficulty begin to evidence itself?" These concepts will become clearer when we walk through an example. However, first fundamental principles on data selection are discussed.

Data Selection

Selection of a data type for measurement of treatment progress should be based on ease of collection, reliability, and the analysis to which the data will be subjected. Further, consideration of what form data collection should take requires that one have a basic understanding of scales of measurement, their characteristics and limitations. A basic understanding can be gained from Hopkins and Glass[3] and the reader is encouraged to review that research. As has been pointed out by others[4,5] the ways in which data can be manipulated are in many respects limited by the scale of measurement. For example, one of the more commonly used scales in rehabilitation is the ordinal scale, in which information is rank ordered so that as one moves up or down the scale, there is more or less of what is being measured. The Functional Independence Measure (FIM) is an example of an ordinal scale, as are the Rappaport Disability Rating and Rancho Scales. In a mathematical sense, data derived from ordinal scales are not appropriate for mathematical or statistical manipulation[4] and caution must be taken should one make such manipulation. While there are methods for conversion of data from ordinal to interval scales of measurement,[6] it should not be automatically assumed that such manipulations are possible.

Selection of a data type for measurement of treatment progress, as noted previously, should be based on ease of collection and reliability. There are numerous options available and the one selected will depend on a number of variables. For the purpose of example, we have selected as a training task learning to shower. Taking a shower is a multistep task and we were interested in whether the patient was independent or dependent at each step and also wanted to be able to summarize daily performance. We selected a Task Analysis Data Sheet (Figure 12–1) because it provides a convenient way of keeping track of training sequence as well as step-by-step performance. The data collected are ordinal in that a patient is or is not dependent. Other data sheets that we have created of this type have a range of levels of independence such as independent, minimum, moderate, and maximal assist. But for this training program, we simply wanted to know whether the patient could or could not execute each step in the task analysis. We next wrote each step on the shower protocol on the Task Analysis Data Sheet. This shower training program was not created solely for this patient but rather was selected from a library of self-care training programs called Treatment Protocols.

Data Collection

We have learned the importance of collecting data as generated. This means that for our shower program we will be scoring each step as independent or dependent as the step is completed. If we were to wait until the end of the shower or some later time to record each score, we would run the risk of inaccuracy. This necessity to collect data as generated is an additional reason for keeping data collection as simple as possible. The first step in data collection is to generate a baseline performance. *Baseline data* refer to those data collected prior to training and give a measure of current performance as well as serving as a foundation against which training performance will be measured. Collection of baseline data is critical in that it serves as a functional assessment of the patient's capabilities in terms of which will be necessary to train the patient to the desired level of independence.

Data Display

While data as they appear on a data sheet can be informative, they are often more readily analyzed if converted to a table or a graph. Our experience has been that a graph is the most easily understood and informative method of data display. On the graph constructed for the shower protocol (Figure 12–2) you will see a number of critical features. The first of these is that we have placed the treatment objective on the graph so that patient, clinician, or payer can quickly see what the objective is. Each treatment objective is written by using the same format such that

Paradigm Health Corporation	PATIENT: Bobby Point	v1.2
DATx® TASK ANALYSIS	WEEK ENDING: 19-DEC	
DATA SHEET	PROTOCOL(S): SHOWER	

INSTRUCTIONS   I = INDEPENDENT

1. STEP refers to each individual component of a skill or task.   D = DEPENDENT
2. STEPS should be completed sequentially.
3. PROMPT LEVEL refers to whether or not the patient required assistance for each step in the task analysis. Circle I if the patient didn't require verbal or physical assistance, circle D if s/he did. SEE PROTOCOL FOR PROMPT HIERARCHY.

STEP	PROMPT LEVEL	STEP	PROMPT LEVEL
1. Turn on water.	ⓘ I I I I I I I I I / D D D D D D D D D D	14. Hang-up towel.	ⓘ I I I I I I I I I / D D D D D D D D D D
2. Regulate temperature.	I I I I I I I I I I / ⒹD D D D D D D D D		I I I I I I I I I I / D D D D D D D D D D
3. Enter shower.	ⓘ I I I I I I I I I / D D D D D D D D D D		I I I I I I I I I I / D D D D D D D D D D
4. Wet hair.	ⓘ I I I I I I I I I / D D D D D D D D D D		I I I I I I I I I I / D D D D D D D D D D
5. Shampoo hair.	I I I I I I I I I I / Ⓓ D D D D D D D D D		I I I I I I I I / D D D D D D D D
6. Rinse hair.	I I I I I I I I I I / Ⓓ D D D D D D D D D		I I I I I I I I / D D D D D D D D
7. Wet body.	ⓘ I I I I I I I I I / D D D D D D D D D D		I I I I I I I I I I / D D D D D D D D D D
8. Wet and soap washcloth.	ⓘ I I I I I / D D D D D D		I I I I I I I I I I / D D D D D D D D D D
9. Wash body.	I I I I I I I / Ⓓ D D D D D D		I I I I I I I I I I / D D D D D D D D D D
10. Rinse body.	ⓘ I I I I I I I I I / D D D D D D D D D D		I I I I I I I I I I / D D D D D D D D D D
11. Turn water off.	ⓘ I I I I I I I I I / D D D D D D D D D D		I I I I I I I I I I / D D D D D D D D D D
12. Exit shower.	ⓘ I I I I I I I I I / D D D D D D D D D D		I I I I I I I I I I / D D D D D D D D D D
13. Dry hair and body.	I I I I I I I I I I / Ⓓ D D D D D D D D D		I I I I I I I I I I / D D D D D D D D D D
DATE	2/4	DATE	
INITIALS	BC	INITIALS	

INITIALS	PRINT FULL NAME	TITLE	INITIALS	PRINT FULL NAME	TITLE

Figure 12–1 Data Sheet. *Source*: Copyright © 1994, Paradigm Health Corporation.

context is specified as are the skill or behavior to be acquired, the performance level, and a stability criterion. We have also drawn a horizontal line that designates the level at which the patient must perform for us to qualify treatment as successful. The patient's performance during baseline is included as well as performance during subsequent training sessions. For the purpose of providing a measure of overall performance, we reported the data as a percentage of steps independent. We could have just as readily reported them as number of steps independent.

Prediction and Control

The area of prediction and control is more related to the concept of knowledge than data; however, the explication of the construct of knowledge is easier to understand in the context of discussing data. We began this chapter with a description of treatment protocols that indicated that each protocol was cross-validated between clinicians specifically in rela-

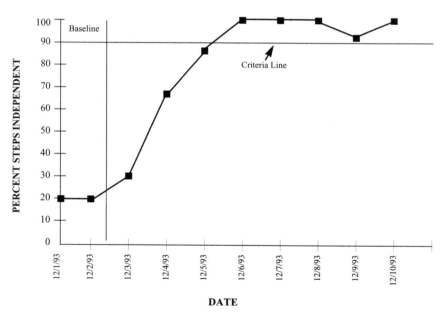

Note: Treatment Objective: During morning activities of daily living, patient will independently complete 90% of shower task, each day, for three consecutive days.

Figure 12–2 Bobby Point Shower Protocol

tion to efficacy as well as resources expended to achieve criterion performance. The shower protocol reflects best demonstrated practice and supplies standards specific to patient progress toward outcome achievement.
This process allows for prediction of the amount of time and resources
needed to achieve the outcome prior to beginning the treatment. It also
allows the clinicians and clinical managers to evaluate *actual* progress
against that which was *predicted.* Variances from the database for similar
patients serve as the foundation for decision making. The decisions may
be to continue as is, revise, or abrogate the plan. The decision that is
made is a reflection of the construct of **knowledge,** in that it reflects the
user's ability to take data, organize them into information, and then use
that information to make decisions. Knowledge builds on itself and thus
the decisions that are made with this particular patient are fed back into
the system that provides the historical data (database) to be used with
subsequent patients. A true knowledge system will allow you to rank
order the importance of the variables that you consider when making a
decision and provide you with a decision based on those rank orderings.
A more detailed analysis of this process will be discussed in the section
on knowledge.

INFORMATION: SYSTEMS AND ORGANIZATION OF DATA

Information and information systems are the foundation of a knowledge-based organization. In order for knowledge to be created and data
to be collected, a system must be in place to organize the process.
Developing an information system that captures data and subsequently
provides information and knowledge is no small task. It requires many
resources, behavioral change, and substantial support from executive and
senior management. Astute managers and executives understand that
more effective capture, management, and use of information are critical
to sustaining and expanding market share.

One approach to developing an information system is to automate
existing processes. An excellent opportunity exists, however, to reinvent
your business consistent with state of the art rehabilitation practices
described in this book. Inching toward this model through incremental
change is not enough for many companies today. Change programs treat
symptoms, not underlying conditions. Companies don't need to change

what is: they need to create what is not. Unfortunately, many executives do not have the courage or see the need to throw away the context they have created.

Like Einstein's thought experiment of riding on a photon of light to see what the world looked like from that perspective, the executive who would master reinvention must journey into a largely unfamiliar and uncomfortable territory, the territory of *being*. Being alters action; context shapes thinking and perception. When one fundamentally alter the context, the foundation on which people construct their understanding of the world, actions are altered accordingly.

The information system a company develops should be flexible and easily accessible by users and should build a knowledge or expert system incrementally from the outset. The flexibility and accessibility of the system will allow users to leverage information when and where it will do the most good and encourage the system's enterprisewide use. Every piece of data entered in the system will allow a company to progress toward information and knowledge.

KNOWLEDGE: ACHIEVING OUTCOMES

Writers on knowledge-based business characterize these enterprises as having six characteristics. They quickly point out that rarely does any one business possess all six characteristics; however, these characteristics can serve as guidelines for developing businesses. A number of these are particularly relevant to outcome-driven rehabilitation. The characteristics are briefly summarized as follows:

1. *The more you use knowledge-based offerings, the smarter they get.* This characteristic refers to systems that feed back information so that better decisions can be made. One example that was given involved the Baldridge award–winning Ritz-Carlton Hotel. If a guest checks into the Ritz-Carlton in Boston and requests hypoallergenic pillows, that customer will find them in her room automatically next time whether she checks into the Ritz-Carlton in Pasadena, California; Hawaii; or Hong Kong. Similarly in the scenario we created at the beginning of the chapter, it follows that once the system is set up, the actual costs, number of treatments necessary to complete the various protocols, targeted outcome that was actually achieved, and eventual outcome level achieved are all fed back into the system to determine whether the predictions were correct. And if

they were not, adjustments can be made in the regression equations to improve subsequent predictions for patients with similar characteristics. As long as the data are collected accurately, each patient added to the system only serves to make the system smarter.

2. *The more you use knowledge-based offerings, the smarter you get.* This characteristic refers to services that enable their users to learn. The example used to illustrate this point is taken from the auto industry. General Motors has a computer aided maintenance system (CAMS). This system is designed to assist novice mechanics in diagnosing and repairing cars. GM noted in the mid-1960s a mechanic only had to know the equivalent of 500 pages of repair manuals to fix any car on the road. Today, the equivalent information would be 500,000 pages of repair manuals. By using the CAMS, the mechanics are smarter because they have access to the knowledge of all other mechanics through this information system. The result is better service to the customer. In our example, *RehaSys* is a repository of knowledge of rehabilitation to which the master clinicians around the country contribute. Imagine the potential utility if we were to have the ten top occupational therapists in the country design a self-care training program for brain injury patients and then had data collected on that protocol by thousands of occupational therapists around the country and had an information system that would organize those data into critical pathways. The results would be a very smart system with smart therapists using the system so that they could do a better job of treating patients.

3. *Knowledge-based products and services adjust to changing circumstances.*This characteristic is particularly representative of smart systems. Davis and Botkin[7] indicated that Goodyear has developed a "smart tire" that contains a microchip that collects and analyzes data about tire pressure. The plan is to have the chip flash a message to the dashboard that states, "Low Tire Pressure — Time for a Pit Stop." The first part of the message conveys information; the second relates knowledge and tells you what to do. Similarly expert systems in rehabilitation can utilize information to alter a course of treatment. For example, using our shower protocol, the database may indicate that if the patient scores as dependent on seven steps or more for six consecutive training sessions, there is a .05 probability that the patient will ever learn the shower sequence. With such data, the occupational therapist can alter the course of treatment and focus on a different functional task to be learned. This is the essence of an expert system

— the collection and organization of data to allow the user to make decisions that can lead to efficient and effective resource utilization.

4. *Knowledge-based businesses can customize their offerings.* This characteristic refers to the fact that knowledge-based business can be responsive to customers' changing needs and idiosyncrasies. One example that was given had to do with new developments in the telecommunication industry. It was pointed out that telephone companies are creating "smart" services that you can create your own distinctive ring so that your best friend knows that it is you. Customization, of course, is not unique to health care. Individualized treatment plans are the norm for rehabilitation services. Individualization, however, can sometimes be used as a justification for not being rigorous in how we develop treatment plans. A knowledge-based approach to rehabilitation allows us to determine first what the norm is for learning a new skill (e.g., the rehabilitation nursing protocol for teaching self-catheterization to a spinal cord injury patient in six training sessions and two follow-ups plus the cost of supplies). Then, the individuation is determined by other predictor variables (e.g., if the patient has a brain injury with a loss of consciousness of 1 day or less, there is no change in the normative training; if the patient has a loss of consciousness of 1–7 days, then the training time is double; if the patient has a loss of consciousness greater than 7 days, self-catheterization is not a realistic outcome goal and should not be incorporated into the treatment plan).

5. *Knowledge-based products and services have relatively short life cycles.* Davis and Botkin point out that patent protections on intellectual property are not nearly as developed as they are on hard technologies; thus, the half-life of proprietary information is short. This phenomenon is even more evident in the field of health care, as it should be. As quickly as treatments, medicines, and therapy approaches are demonstrated to be efficacious and then validated, they need to get out into the public domain. However, it should not stop there and this is where knowledge-based systems can perhaps have their greatest impact. The value the knowledge-based system has in this situation is to provide a mechanism by which results from the treatment implementation can be fed back to lead to further improvements and refinements in the treatments or even further identify for whom the treatment is effective and for whom it is not. Throughout the history of rehabilitation, efforts of this type have been attempted with more or less success. The most successful have

been the Model Systems Grants for spinal cord injury and brain injury. Among the flaws in these approaches have been system design and the nature and quantity of the data being collected. The data that can be analyzed from these systems tend to reflect trends and not provide specificity around how clinicians should be treating patients differently. The FIM data from the Uniform Data System (UDS) are another large source of information that will prove to be invaluable in the future.[8] Again, this system was designed to provide information on trends and serve as a baseline against which rehabilitation facilities can compare their overall performance on an ongoing basis. It was not designed to be a smart system that would help a program to improve. A knowledge-based system, as was pointed out previously, gets smarter the more you use it and makes the end user smarter as well. As a consequence, it may have a short half-life because it is constantly reinventing itself. For example, in our shower protocol, let's say it has been replicated 120 times with an average number of sessions to reach criterion being 8. In 60 of those cases, the average number of sessions was 10. These were the cases with a length of unconsciousness of greater than 7 days. In the other 60 cases, the average number of training sessions was 6. These cases had a length of unconsciousness of less than or equal to 7 days. Additionally, on these cases, the patient was independent on 3 of the 13 steps at the onset of treatment. Therefore, on the basis of this information, we were able to improve the efficiency of the service delivery and improve our knowledge of self-care training of brain injury patients. Finally, we were able to reengineer a treatment protocol. The next 120 replications of this protocol may lead to further improvements.

6. *Knowledge-based businesses enable customers to act in real time.* This is perhaps one of the most exciting possibilities to evolve from knowledge-based businesses and services. A couple of interesting examples of this were given in the Davis and Botkin article. The first noted that automakers are preparing to deliver AAA Triptik-type information electronically in vehicles in real time. Drivers will be given information regarding what highways to take and what hotels and other hot spots are on the route. This information will be delivered in real time in the comfort of your vehicle. Additionally, this information will be continually updated with traffic reports displayed on a dashboard screen. Currently, Xerox provides preventive maintenance for some of its large machines with a built-in modem that automatically calls for field service. In a few of the larger

medical schools around the country, physicians are doing construct and concurrent validation studies with personal assistive devices (PADs). These are small hand-held computers similar to the Apple Newton computer that allow the physician to input the patient's symptoms and any other diagnostic data and then give a read-out of the patient's diagnosis and a specification of what the most clinically accepted treatment regimen would be for that particular patient. Just as our opening scenario indicates, this approach is not too distant in the future for the field of of rehabilitation as well. It is entirely conceivable that a coordinated interdisciplinary team assessment could be completed and the data inputted into a system that would prescribe the type of rehabilitation services needed, the functional goals to be accomplished, the treatment protocols indicated to achieve the goals, and the treatment length that would be required to complete the treatment protocols. Haig et al[8] and their work on the single-visit assessment provide a good starting point for the single-coordinated-assessment approach. The development and implementation of data-based protocols are being done on state-of-the-art rehabilitation programs around the country and are discussed in the chapters by Haffey, Bryant, and Evans in this text. What we are not doing is integrating the entire process and the feedback of the data back into the information systems in order to create smarter protocols and treatments. A knowledge-based organization does this.

Davis and Botkin, in summarizing their article, indicate that the development of knowledge-based businesses is a reflection of an even greater transformation in our society in terms of knowledge and learning. Knowledge is doubling every 7 years. For companies to remain competitive and workers to stay employable, learning has to be continuous. Garvin[9] in his much-quoted article, "Building a Learning Organization," uses the terms "learning organization," "knowledge-creating organization," and "knowledge-based organization" synonymously. He defines a learning organization as "an organization skilled in creating, acquiring, and transferring knowledge, and at modifying its behavior to reflect new knowledge and insights." He then goes on to point out that learning organizations are characterized by five principal activities: (1) systematic problem solving, (2) experimentation with new approaches, (3) learning from their own experience and past history, (4) learning from the experiences and best practices of others, and (5) transferring knowledge quickly and efficiently throughout the organization.

When I think about what rehabilitation is, it encompasses these principles better than most types of fields or businesses. Our challenge today is taking the time to be careful and rigorous in what we are doing so that we can build smarter rehabilitation organizations for tomorrow.

REFERENCES

1. Peters MD, Gluck M, McCormick M. Behavior rehabilitation of the challenging client in less restrictive settings. *Brain Injury.* 1992;6(4):299–314.

2. Pace GM, Nau PA. Behavior analysis in brain injury rehabilitation: training staff to develop, implement, and evaluate behavior change programs. In: *Staff Development and Clinical Intervention in Brain Injury Rehabilitation.* Gaithersburg, Md:Aspen Publishers, Inc; 105–127.

3. Hopkins KD and Glass GV. Basic Statistics for the Behavioral Sciences. Englewood Cliffs, NJ:Prentice-Hall Inc.; 10–13.

4. Merbitz C, Morris J, Grip, JC. Ordinal scales and foundations of misinference. *Arch Phys Med Rehabil.* 1989;70:308–312.

5. McLean A, Cardenas DD, Haselkorn JK, Peters MD. Cognitive psychopharmacology. *NeuroRehabilitation.* 1993;3(2):1–14.

6. Wright BD and Linacre JM. Observations are always ordinal; measurements, however, must be interval. *Arch Phys Med Rehabil.* 1989;70:857–860.

7. Davis S, Botkin J. The coming of knowledge-based business. *Harvard Bus Rev.* September-October 1994: 165–170.

8. Haig AJ, Nagy A, LeBreck D, et al. Patient-oriented rehabilitation planning in a single visit: first-year review of the Quick Program. *Arch Phys Med Rehabil.* 1994;75:172–176.

9. Garvin D. Building a learning organization. *Harvard Business Review.* July-August 1993:78–91.

Index

paradigm rehabilitation outcome
levels, 158
physiologic instability, 47–48, 58–59
physiologic maintenance, 49–51
physiologic stability, 48–49, 57–67
primary functional goals, 50
productivity activity, 51–52
Outcome–oriented approach
critical pathways in, 157
documentation system in, 157,
165–174
emphasis in, 134
enterprise for. See Enterprise for
outcome–based rehabilitation
example of, 133
focus in, 133
organizational factors, 148–149
outcome based on evaluation, 154
and outcomes management, 148–149
outcome tracking system in, 175
patient–centered assessment in, 157,
159–164
people challenges in, 134–137
process challenges in, 137–142
rehabilitation goals in, 154
rehabilitation plan in, 155–156
senior management role in, 149–150
stress related to, 136–137
system challenges in, 142–145
team communication in, 175–178
training of staff, 150–156
Outcomes
for acute rehabilitation setting, 70
areas examined by researchers, 70
continuum of patient–specific
outcomes, 52–54
definition of, 69
in delivery of results–oriented
rehabilitation, 54–56
effects on rehabilitation system, 44–46
global outcome, 44
outcome levels, 44
patient–specific outcomes, 44, 65–66
planning for outcome, 64–67

Outcomes management, 33–36
continuous quality improvement,
114–116
as dynamic process, 111, 113
generic measures, 34–35
organizational factors in, 148–149
outcome validation system, 113–114
program evaluation, 113
public disclosure of data, 35–36
quality assurance, 117–118
risk adjustment in, 34
role of, 33
scope of, 33–34
senior management, role of, 149–151
Outcome tracking, in outcome–oriented
approach, 175
Outcome validation system, 113–114
outcomes in, 114

P

Partnership assessment scale, 285
Partnerships, in outcome–based
sales/marketing, 281–283
Past, and transformational management,
250–253
Patient, use of term, 135
Patient Evaluation and Conference
System (PECS), 33–34, 139
Patient–specific outcomes, types of, 44,
65–66
Payer–driven system
health care, 4–5, 22–24
and medical rehabilitation, 36
Payers of medical rehabilitation, 14–16
managed care, impact of, 16–17
Medicaid, 15
Medicare, 15
overview of, 14
private health insurance, 15–16
and prospective payment system,
16–17
Perfect competition, 25
Perfect knowledge, 27–28